MW00744375

ALZHEIMER'S: THINGS A NURSE NEEDS TO KNOW

First Edition

By
Joan Cagley-Knight, MSN, ARNP

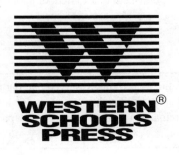

WESTERN SCHOOLS PRESS ®

21 Bristol Drive
South Easton, MA 02375
1-800-618-1670

ABOUT THE AUTHOR

Joan Cagley-Knight, MSN, ARNP, is a registered nurse specialist in field operations with Health Quality Assurance, Agency for Health Care Administration, Area 8, Fort Myers, FL. She holds a Master of Science in Nursing from the University of South Florida, Tampa, FL and a Master of Arts in Counseling from the University of Northern Iowa in Cedar Falls, IA. For 10 years Ms. Cagley-Knight was a nursing instructor at Hawkeye Community College in Waterloo, IA. She is also a certified federal/state surveyor for long term care facilities and the former director of educational services at a national educational video company where she wrote and/or produced 50 educational video tapes for long term care and home health staff use.

ABOUT THE SUBJECT MATTER EXPERT

Suzanne Doyle Friedman, MS, RN, a psychotherapist in private practice, was the Program Coordinator for the Geriatric Mental Health Designated Bed Project, a collaborative nursing home project between the University of Maryland School of Nursing and the Mental Hygiene Administration, Department of Health and Mental Hygiene, State of Maryland. She has experience in program development and implementation, administration/management, and consultation in the long-term care arena. Ms Friedman's area of interest is in programmatic issues in the care of cognitively impaired elderly. She has master's level preparation in both gerontological and psychiatric-mental health nursing, with functional expertise in both administration and clinical specialization and is currently pursuing her PhD in family studies.

Copy Editor: Barbara Halliburton, PhD

Indexer: Sylvia Coates

Typesetter: Kathy Johnson

Western Schools' courses are designed to provide nursing professionals with the educational information they need to enhance their career development. The information provided within these course materials is the result of research and consultation with prominent nursing and medical authorities and is, to the best of our knowledge, current and accurate. However, the courses and course materials are provided with the understanding that Western Schools is not engaged in offering legal, nursing, medical, or other professional advice.

Western Schools' courses and course materials are not meant to act as a substitute for seeking out professional advice or conducting individual research. When the information provided in the courses and course materials is applied to individual circumstances, all recommendations must be considered in light of the uniqueness pertaining to each situation.

Western Schools' course materials are intended solely for *your* use and *not* for the benefit of providing advice or recommendations to third parties. Western Schools devoids itself of any responsibility for adverse consequences resulting from the failure to seek nursing, medical, or other professional advice. Western Schools further devoids itself of any responsibility for updating or revising any programs or publications presented, published, distributed, or sponsored by Western Schools unless otherwise agreed to as part of an individual purchase contract.

ISBN: 1-57801-012-8

COPYRIGHT© 1997—Western Schools, Inc. All Rights Reserved. No part(s) of this material may be reprinted, reproduced, transmitted, stored in a retrieval system, or otherwise utilized, in any form or by any means electronic or mechanical, including photocopying or recording, now existing or hereinafter invented, nor may any part of this course be used for teaching without the written permission from the publisher and author.

IMPORTANT: Read these instructions *BEFORE* proceeding!

Enclosed with your course book you will find the FasTrax® answer sheet. Use this form to answer all the final exam questions that appear in this course book. If you are completing more than one course, be sure to write your answers on the appropriate answer sheet. Full instructions and complete grading details are printed on the FasTrax instruction sheet, also enclosed with your order. Please review them before starting. *If you are mailing your answer sheet(s) to Western Schools, we recommend you make a copy as a backup.*

ABOUT THIS COURSE

A "Pretest" is provided with each course to test your current knowledge base regarding the subject matter contained within this course. Your "Final Exam" is a multiple choice examination. **You will find the exam questions at the end of each chapter.** Some smaller hour courses include the exam at the end of the book.

In the event the course has less than 100 questions, mark your answers to the questions in the course book and leave the remaining answer boxes on the FasTrax answer sheet blank. **Use a <u>black pen</u> to fill in your answer sheet.**

A PASSING SCORE

You must score 70% or better in order to pass this course and receive your Certificate of Completion. Should you fail to achieve the required score, we will send you an additional FasTrax answer sheet so that you may make a second attempt to pass the course. Western Schools will allow you three chances to pass the same course...*at no extra charge!* After three failed attempts to pass the same course, your file will be closed.

RECORDING YOUR HOURS

Please monitor the time it takes to complete this course using the handy log sheet on the other side of this page. See below for transferring study hours to the course evaluation.

COURSE EVALUATIONS

In this course book you will find a short evaluation about the course you are soon to complete. This information is vital to providing the school with feedback on this course. The course evaluation answer section is in the lower right hand corner of the FasTrax answer sheet marked "Evaluation" with answers marked 1–25. Your answers are important to us, please take five minutes to complete the evaluation.

On the back of the FasTrax instruction sheet there is additional space to make any comments about the course, the school, and suggested new curriculum. Please mail the FasTrax instruction sheet, with your comments, back to Western Schools in the envelope provided with your course order.

TRANSFERRING STUDY TIME

Upon completion of the course, transfer the total study time from your log sheet to question #25 in the Course Evaluation. The answers will be in ranges, please choose the proper hour range that best represents your study time. You MUST log your study time under question #25 on the course evaluation.

EXTENSIONS

You have 2 years from the date of enrollment to complete this course. A six (6) month extension may be purchased. If after 30 months from the original enrollment date you do not complete the course, *your file will be closed and no certificate can be issued.*

CHANGE OF ADDRESS?

In the event you have moved during the completion of this course please call our student services department at 1-800-618-1670 and we will update your file.

A GUARANTEE YOU'LL GIVE HIGH HONORS TO

If any continuing education course fails to meet your expectations or if you are not satisfied in any manner, for any reason, you may return it for an exchange or a refund (less shipping and handling) within 30 days. Software, video and audio courses must be returned unopened.

Thank you for enrolling at Western Schools!

WESTERN SCHOOLS
P.O. Box 1930
Brockton, MA 02303
(800) 618-1670

ALZHEIMER'S: THINGS A NURSE NEEDS TO KNOW

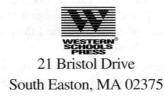

21 Bristol Drive
South Easton, MA 02375

Please use this log to total the number of hours you spend reading the text and taking the final examination (use 50-min hours).

Date	Hours Spent
_____	_____
_____	_____
_____	_____
_____	_____
_____	_____
_____	_____
_____	_____
_____	_____
_____	_____
_____	_____
_____	_____
_____	_____
_____	_____

TOTAL

Please log your study hours with submission of your final exam. To log your study time, fill in the appropriate circle under question 25 of the FasTrax® answer sheet under the "Evaluation" section.

PLEASE LOG YOUR STUDY HOURS WITH SUBMISSION OF YOUR FINAL EXAM. Please choose which best represents the total study hours it took to complete this 12 hour course.

A. less than 7 hours

B. 7–9 hours

C. 10–13 hours

D. greater than 13 hours

ALZHEIMER'S: THINGS A NURSE NEEDS TO KNOW

WESTERN SCHOOLS
CONTINUING EDUCATION EVALUATION

Instructions: Mark your answers to the following questions with a black pen on the "Evaluation" section of your FasTrax® answer sheet provided with this course. You should not return this sheet. Please use the scale below to rate the following statements:

A Agree Strongly	**C Disagree Somewhat**
B Agree Somewhat	**D Disagree Strongly**

The course content met the following education objectives:

1. Described what Alzheimer's disease is and what it is not.

2. Described the role of the nurse in supporting family or staff caregivers of individuals with Alzheimer's disease and described how to help caregivers make choices about available types of care taking into account the financial and legal consequences of these decisions.

3. Described common therapeutic approaches to manage the behavioral symptoms of demented individuals and how to incorporate them into nursing practice.

4. Described the nursing process, including best practice interventions, for multidisciplinary concerns of individuals with Alzheimer's.

5. Explained the rationale for using alternatives to physical and chemical restraints to manage behaviors and the appropriate nursing management of behaviors that may occur when caring for an individual with Alzheimer's disease, including wandering, resisting care, sleeping problems and catastrophic reactions.

6. The content of this course was relevant to the objectives.

7. This offering met my professional education needs.

8. The information in this offering is relevant to my professional work setting.

9. The course was generally well written and the subject matter explained thoroughly? (If no please explain on the back of the FasTrax instruction sheet.)

10. The content of this course was appropriate for home study.

11. The final examination was well written and at an appropriate level for the content of the course.

Please complete the following research questions in order to help us better meet your educational needs. Pick the ONE answer which is most appropriate.

12. Why do you choose home study to fulfill some or all of your license renewal requirements?

    A. Price   C. Permanent reference material

    B. Convenience to study when you want   D. Large variety of course selections

13. Why did you select Western Schools as your Continuing Education provider?

    A. Broad list of professional accreditations   C. Reputation for quality, up-to-date course materials

    B. Service/Delivery   D. Price

14. How did you fulfill the majority of your CE requirement the time just before this Western Schools order?

    A. Western Schools   C. Seminars or in-house lectures

    B. Another home study provider   D. No previous occasion

15. Which answer best describes the portion of your total Continuing Education hours that were completed by home study during your last renewal?
    A. All
    B. Half to more than half
    C. Less than half
    D. None

16. Are you reimbursed for your Continuing Education hours, and if so, by what dollar percentage?
    A. All
    B. Half to more than half
    C. Less than half
    D. None

17. What is your work status?
    A. Full-time employment
    B. Part-time employment
    C. Per diem/Temporary employment
    D. Inactive/Retired

18. For your LAST renewal did you take more Continuing Education contact hours than required by your state, if so, how many?
    A. 1–15 hours
    B. 16–30 hours
    C. 31 or more hours
    D. No, I only take the state required minimum

19. Do you usually exceed the contact hours required for your state license renewal, if so, why?
    A. Yes, I have more than one state license
    B. Yes, to meet additional special association Continuing Education requirements
    C. Yes, for professional self-interest/cross-training
    D. No, I only take the state required minimum

20. What nursing shift do you most commonly work?
    A. Morning Shift (Any shift starting after 3:00am or before 11:00am)
    B. Day/Afternoon Shift (Any shift starting after 11:00am or before 7:00pm)
    C. Night Shift (Any shift starting after 7:00pm or before 3:00am)
    D. I work rotating shifts

21. What was the SINGLE most important reason you chose this course?
    A. Low Price
    B. New or Newly revised course
    C. High interest/Required course topic
    D. Number of Contact Hours Needed

22. Where do you work? (If your place of employment is not listed below, please leave this question blank.)
    A. Hospital
    B. Medical Clinic/Group Practice/ HMO/Office setting
    C. Long Term Care/Rehabilitation Facility/Nursing Home
    D. Home Health Care Agency

23. Which field do you specialize in?
    A. Medical/Surgical
    B. Geriatrics
    C. Pediatrics/Neonatal
    D. Other

24. For your last renewal, how many months BEFORE your license expiration date did you order your course materials?
    A. 1–3 months
    B. 4–6 months
    C. 7–12 months
    D. Greater than 12 months

25. **PLEASE LOG YOUR STUDY HOURS WITH SUBMISSION OF YOUR FINAL EXAM.** Please choose which best represents the total study hours it took to complete this 12 hour course.
    A. less than 7 hours
    B. 7–9 hours
    C. 10–13 hours
    D. greater than 13 hours

CONTENTS

PRETEST

Begin by taking the pretest. Compare your answers on the pretest to the answer key (located in the back of the book). Circle those test items that you missed. The pretest answer key indicates the course chapters where the content of that question is discussed.

Next, read each chapter. Focus special attention on the chapters where you made incorrect answer choices. Exam questions are provided at the end of each chapter so that you can assess your progress and understanding of the material.

1. Which of the following statements reflects the relationship between Alzheimer's disease and aging?

   A. Memory loss is an expected part of aging.

   B. Fewer than 3 million persons in the United States currently have Alzheimer's disease.

   C. Alzheimer's disease is only one type of dementia that can occur with aging.

   D. Dementia occurs with most diseases as a person ages.

2. Guidelines for interviewing a confused older person include which of the following?

   A. Move slowly, but speak quickly before attention is lost.

   B. Do not call the person by his or her name if doing so is distracting.

   C. Conduct the interview in a public area if the person is confrontational.

   D. Sit at the same level as the person being interviewed and use a calm, level tone of voice.

3. What percent of Americans who became 65 years old in 1990 will spend time as a resident in a nursing home?

   A. 5–15%

   B. 25–30%

   C. 40–45%

   D. 50–60%

4. Which of the following is most important when a caregiver is choosing a nursing home?

   A. Caregiver's preference

   B. Location

   C. Cost

   D. Food

5. The purpose of exploring therapeutic approaches to caring for demented patients is to do which of the following?

   A. Overcome memory loss and agitation.

   B. Provide a framework for attempts to understand what behavioral signs mean.

   C. Challenge nurses to look for other ways of caring for demented patients.

   D. Realize what facilities or agencies may base nursing care on.

6. Which therapeutic approach has improved depression in patients with dementia?

    A. Reality orientation

    B. Validation therapy

    C. Organizational structure of the environment

    D. Reminiscence

7. Which of the following are two communication problems experienced by many patients with Alzheimer's disease?

    A. Speaking slowly and thinking slowly

    B. Difficulty expressing wishes to others and inability to understand what is being said by others

    C. Trying to find the right word for something and ignoring what is not understood

    D. Withdrawing from social situations and laughing inappropriately

8. What is the most specific indicator of nutritional status in the elderly?

    A. Wandering

    B. Obesity

    C. Change in body weight

    D. Serum albumin level

9. Who has typically initiated restraining an elderly hospitalized patient?

    A. The doctor

    B. The nursing assistant

    C. The patient's family

    D. The nurse

10. What happens to the levels of fat and water in the body as a person ages?

    A. Little or no change

    B. Less water, more fat

    C. More water, less fat

    D. More fat and more water

CHAPTER 1

ALZHEIMER'S DISEASE: WHAT IT IS AND IS NOT

CHAPTER OBJECTIVE

After completing this chapter, the reader will be able to describe what Alzheimer's disease is and what it is not.

LEARNING OBJECTIVES

After studying this chapter, the reader will be able to

1. Recognize various types of progressive degenerative dementia.

2. Specify the incidence of Alzheimer's disease.

3. Compare normal changes in the central nervous system (CNS) that occur with aging with pathophysiological changes that occur in Alzheimer's disease.

4. Differentiate between indications of dementia, depression, and delirium.

5. Specify the four *A's* that indicate areas of loss in cognitive impairment.

6. Contrast the early, middle, and late stages of Alzheimer's disease.

INTRODUCTION

How will we age? Each of us wonders about this question. Probably the best way to judge the answer is to examine how we are handling our "middle age." We tend to become "more of ourselves" as we grow older. Someone who has always been outspoken and opinionated or fun loving and sociable most likely will act the same way when he or she is older. It is important to recognize that confusion, memory loss, and other behavioral problems should not be an expected part of aging.

Consider the poem "I Can't Remember":

Just a line to say I'm living,

that I'm not among the dead,

though I'm getting more forgetful

and mixed up in my head.

    I got used to my arthritis,

    to my dentures I'm resigned.

    I can manage my bifocals,

    but, God, I miss my mind.

For sometimes I can't remember

when I stand at the foot of the stairs,

if I must go up for something

or have just come down from there.

    And, before the fridge so often,

    my poor mind is filled with doubt,

    have I just put food away,

    or have I come to take some out?

And, there are times when it is dark,

with my nightcap on my head,

I don't know if I'm retiring

or just getting out of bed.

So if it's my turn to write you,

there's no need for getting sore—

I may think I've written

and don't want to be a bore!

So remember that I love you

and wish that you were near,

but now it's nearly mail time,

so I must say "Good-bye, Dear."

P.S. Here I stand beside the mailbox

with a face so very red—

Instead of mailing you my letter,

I have opened it instead!

Anonymous

Currently, between 3 million and 4 million persons in the United States have Alzheimer's disease. Consequently, although Alzheimer's disease or dementia might not affect every person, it will continue to be a significant issue in caring for the elderly. After age 65 years, the percentage of affected persons with dementia or Alzheimer's disease approximately doubles with each decade of life that passes (McNeil, 1995).

This chapter examines the types of dementia and describes tools to help differentiate between dementia, depression, and delirium. Recognizing the underlying disease is vital. The chapter reviews the components of the clinical diagnosis of Alzheimer's disease and nursing interventions to facilitate diagnosis. It also describes normal aging, the pathophysiology of dementia, and stages of Alzheimer's disease.

TYPES OF COGNITIVE IMPAIRMENT

Alzheimer's disease is not a new phenomenon. However, before the past 20 years, little was known about it. The ancient Greeks and Romans described signs and symptoms similar to those of Alzheimer's disease. Even Shakespeare noted, in the 16th century, that in extreme old age, the signs of second childishness or mere oblivion were known and recognized. In the early 1900s, during an autopsy of a former patient, Dr. Alois Alzheimer detected the signs of the brain disease that is named after him. Although when the patient was alive, Dr. Alzheimer thought that she was experiencing a mental illness, during the autopsy, he found dense deposits outside and around the nerve cells in her brain. These deposits are now called neuritic plaques. Inside the cells he found neurofibrillary tangles or twisted threads of fiber. Detection of plaques and tangles at autopsy remain the best way to diagnose Alzheimer's disease.

Three types of illness affect the mental health of the elderly: dementia, delirium, and depression *(Table 1-1)*.

DEMENTIA

Dementia is an organic mental disorder characterized by a loss or impairment in mental functioning or cognition. The loss in the ability to think and reason is manifested as changes in behavior and intellectual functioning. The changes affect memory, verbal skills, math skills, and spatial-visual perceptions. The term dementia is accepted by the medical community and families as being less judgmental than other more outdated terms such as organic brain disease and senile dementia.

Approximately 50% of dementias are classified as Alzheimer's dementia, 10–20% are due to vascular disorders such as multi-infarct dementia, and another 20% may be a combination of Alzheimer's and multi-infarct dementias. Other less common progressive degenerative dementias include the following:

• Korsakoff's psychosis or syndrome related to chronic alcoholism and vitamin E deficiency

• Parkinson's disease

TABLE 1-1
Comparison of Depression, Dementia, and Delirium

	Depression	Dementia	Delirium
Onset	Uncertain date of onset—slow, uneven progression over weeks	Uncertain date of onset—slow, even progression over months or years	Precise date of onset—develops abruptly, often at night
Duration	Generally self-limited, reversed with therapy or ECT, can be chronic	Chronic and irreversible	Usually acute, varies with cause and effective treatment, chronic if untreated
Mood	Stable, constantly withdrawn, apathetic, hopelessness	Panic states, rapid sadness to happiness, fluctuates from apathetic to outgoing	Anxiety, restlessness, aggressiveness
Self-image	Poor, makes self-derogative statements, worthlessness, feels empty	No self-deprecation	No self-deprecation, misidentification
Course	Progressive, present for many months or years	Progressive, present for many years	Nonprogressive, short duration
Memory	Complains of memory loss, forgets parts of experience	Attempts to hide memory loss, forgets whole experience	Does not note memory loss, forgets most of experience
Consciousness	Rarely altered consciousness	Rarely altered consciousness	Fluctuating consciousness
Diurnal pattern	Often worse in the morning, better as the day goes on	Worse later in day or when fatigued	No relation to time of day or fatigue
Level of awareness	Aware of, exaggerates disability, focuses on self, despondent	Unaware of or minimizes disability, declines with time, lucid intervals early in disease	No awareness of disability, awareness fluctuates hallucinates, delusions, appears frightened, dazed look, lucid intervals
Alcohol, drugs	Many use alcohol or drugs	Rarely abuses drugs	Common with situational changes, may be drug induced
Mental competence **Self-care capacity**	Basically unimpaired, little loss of intellect	Loss of intellectual abilities, abstract thinking poor	Clouding of consciousness, slow thinking may be drawn or accelerated
Physical illness or drug toxicity	Generally able, motivation decreased	Generally unable	Usually unable
	Usually absent, coincides often with a loss	Often absent, especially in primary degenerative dementia	Usually present
Sleep/wake cycle	Varies from insomnia to lengthy sleep patterns	Fragmented sleep; erratic sleep and rest patterns	Always disrupted; often drowsiness during the day, insomnia at night

Reprinted with permission of Lippincott-Raven Publishers from Staab, A. S., & Lyles, M. F. (1990). *Manual of geriatric nursing.* Glenview, IL: Scott, Foresman/Little, Brown Higher Education. ECT = electroconvulsive therapy.

- Huntington's chorea

- Pick's disease, a rare disease clinically similar to Alzheimer's disease

- Creutzfeldt-Jakob disease, a slow-acting viral infection influenced by a genetic predisposition

- AIDS-related dementia (10% of patients with AIDS are more than 50 years old, and dementia can be a sign in any patient with AIDS)

DELIRIUM

Acute and reversible dementias with a number of known causes are referred to as delirium. The causes of delirium appear to lie outside the CNS. These conditions are not chronic and are potentially reversible. Delirium is often precipitated by a physical illness manifested as a psychiatric complication. Extreme sleepiness, lethargy, or partial consciousness or hallucinations, delusions, and excitability can be indications of acute states of delirium. In some instances, patients have a mixture of these features.

Unfortunately, transient delirium is common in elderly hospitalized patients, at the time of surgery, and during other periods of enforced sedentary status. It is important for nurses to look for underlying causes of delirium, including pharmaceutical agents. Nurses should be aware of what medications or combinations of either prescription or over-the-counter medications their patients are taking. Sensory deficits (e.g., losses in vision or hearing) can mimic delirium. Delirium can also be due to metabolic disorders, such as hypothyroidism, diabetes, and nutritional deficiencies, which can be detected by laboratory tests.

Common causes of delirium include minor problems, such as rectal impaction or bladder infections, and alcohol abuse or overuse. In most instances, delirium can be treated by treating the underlying medical problem. These widespread causes must be ruled out before a condition can be accepted as irreversible.

DEPRESSION

The incidence of depression in persons more than 65 years old may be as high as 10–15% (Hendric & Crossett, 1990). Like delirium and dementia, depression is not a normal part of aging. Many elderly patients who are depressed have typical signs and symptoms of affective illnesses:

- Depressed mood

- Weight loss or gain

- Changes in appetite

- Inability to sleep or too much sleeping

- Fatigue or loss of energy

- Lowered interest in pleasurable activities

- Low self-esteem

- Inability to concentrate or make decisions

- Anxiety

Older persons who are depressed may not complain about mood changes. Other less typical indications of depression are cognitive loss, pain syndromes, and alcohol abuse (McCollough, 1991).

Depression is a brain disorder of biological origin and is one of the most treatable, and possibly undertreated, diseases of the elderly. Depression occurs in 15–30% of patients with Alzheimer's disease, usually in the early stages. Often depression occurs along with other dementing illnesses such as Parkinson's disease and multi-infract dementia.

In addition, medications used to treat other medical illnesses common in the elderly can cause depression. These include antihypertensives, antiparkinsonians, narcotic analgesics, sedative-hypnotics, corticosteroids, and multiple drugs used in combinations. Nurses should be suspicious of any multiple drug combinations, including over-the-counter drugs, that may have psychotropic effects. Although treatment of depression will not affect the cognitive function of demented elderly patients, their functional independence and quality of life almost always improve.

CLINICAL DIAGNOSIS

The importance of differentiating dementia, delirium, and depression cannot be overemphasized. These three illnesses, which are manifested by cognitive, emotional, and behavioral signs and symptoms, are extremely common in health care facilities, hospitals, and nursing homes and in all areas of nursing, including occupational health, medical offices or clinics, and home health care. The price society pays is a concern, because services designed for and needed by the elderly are increasing rapidly. The estimated annual cost of Alzheimer's disease is $80 billion to $90 billion. This number includes the costs of lost productivity and the costs of care. According to a study in California (Rice, Fox, & Max, 1993), care for a patient with Alzheimer's disease costs *$47,000/year,* whether the person lives in a nursing home or at home.

Because treatment for depression, delirium, and dementia depends on recognizing the underlying disease, accurate assessment of a patient's illness is imperative. Nurses are in a unique position to observe and document changes in status, whether cognitive, emotional, functional or a combination of these. Dementias are physical illnesses, but the manifestations are behavioral. As a person loses control of self and his or her environment, signs occur, such as outbursts of anger; easy annoyance; and aggressive behavior, both physical and verbal. As the disease progresses, other common behavioral problems may occur, including wandering, resisting care, yelling, rummaging through others' belongings, and hostile actions toward caregivers. The increasingly severe behavioral indications are what bring families to the attention of health care providers. The progression of the dementia can vary as the disease proceeds *(Table 1-2).*

Another way of looking at cognitive impairment that has been helpful for health care providers is to recognize the four *A's,* which indicate areas of loss:

1. **Agnosia:** inability to recognize familiar faces, objects, or surroundings. Patients see and hear with acuity but may interpret inaccurately. They may not recognize familiar faces, may not distinguish where they are, and may not realize what belongs to them or to others. Some eventually may not recognize themselves in a mirror.

2. **Amnesia:** loss of the ability to learn new information that appears as forgetfulness. Behaviors thought of as combativeness or resisting care often are due to frustration with forgetting information, repeated questioning, and not being able to find misplaced objects. Well-meaning reward systems intended to change these behaviors may backfire because the new system cannot be learned.

3. **Aphasia:** difficulty in comprehending or expressing language. Patients who are aphasic may be unable to follow directions, express their needs, or converse with another person. Frustration with their inability to express needs and wants can lead to withdrawal and anger. As a result, they may be labeled difficult or moody rather than aphasic.

4. **Apraxia:** loss of ability to perform learned motor skills such as how to open a door, how to dress, or how to use utensils for eating. When a person no longer remembers what a shower or a bathroom is for or how to use it, the sight, smell, and temperature of the room can be terrifying.

Understanding that the four *A's* are neurological losses that a patient is experiencing can help in planning care and in deciding what aspects of the patient's environment may need to be changed or new approaches to be tried.

According to the fourth revised edition of

TABLE 1-2
Characteristic Progression of Alzheimer's Disease: Global Deterioration Scale

Stage	Characteristics	Diagnosis	Duration (avg)	Mood change*
1 Normality	No subjective or objective complaints	Normal adult	50–75 yr	None
2 Forgetfulness	Subjective deficits in word finding, locating objects	Normal, aged adult	15 yr	Concern
3 Early confusional	Difficulty in handling complex occupational tasks	Compatible with incipient Alzheimer's disease	7 yr	Anxiety
4 Late confusional	Needs assistance in complex tasks, such as handling finances, planning holiday meals	Mild Alzheimer's disease	2 yr	Flattening of affect; denial, emotional withdrawal and sometimes tearfulness
5 Early dementia	Can no longer function independently; e.g., needs assistance in choosing proper attire	Moderate Alzheimer's disease	18 mo	Increase in flattening of affect; sometimes anger and/or tearfulness
6 Middle dementia; substage A	Needs assistance dressing	Moderately severe Alzheimer's disease	5 mo	Agitation and psychotic symptoms
substage B	Needs assistance bathing, adjusting water temperature		5 mo	
substage C	Needs assistance in mechanics of toileting, brushing teeth		5 mo	
substage D	Urinary incontinence		4 mo	
substage E	Fecal incontinence		10 mo	
7 Late dementia; substage A	Speech ability limited to a half-dozen intelligible words	Severe Alzheimer's disease	1 yr	Pathologic passivity
substage B	Intelligible vocabulary limited to one word		18 mo	
substage C	Ability to walk is lost		1 yr	
substage D	Ability to sit up is lost		1 yr	
substage E	Ability to smile is lost		18 mo	
substage F	Ability to hold up head is lost		Survival from this point is variable	

*The patient's change in mood is less consistent in the evolution of the disease.

Reprinted with permission from Reisberg, B., Ferris, S. H., Leon, M. J., & Crook, T. (1982). The Global Deterioration Scale for assessment of primary degenerative dementia. *American Journal of Psychiatry, 139,* 1136–1139.

Diagnostic and Statistical Manual of Mental Disorders (American Psychiatric Association, 1994), a variety of changes in intellectual functioning are associated with the normal process of aging. The true nature and extent of these changes and whether they should be considered part of normal functional loss with age remain controversial:

> The diagnosis of dementia is warranted only if there is demonstrable evidence of memory impairment that, along with the other features of dementia, is of sufficient severity to interfere with social or occupational functioning. Dementia is not synonymous with aging. (p. 106)

The persistence of signs of impaired intellectual function over a period of months, in a relatively stable form, suggests dementia rather than delirium *(Tables 1-3A and 1-3B)*. Exclusion of all other specific causes of dementia is vital. Other causes can be detected by obtaining an extensive history, by physical examination, and by laboratory tests *(Table 1-4)*. Any specific tests indicated by the patient's history and psychological evaluation should be done. It is essential to assess patients for concurrent illnesses that can mimic Alzheimer's disease or dementia.

As much as possible, the patient and the patient's family should be involved in obtaining a comprehensive history. The history should include information on the patient's social, cultural, ethnic, and familial background. The information should be gathered over the course of several interviews to encourage as much participation as possible by the person who is the focus of the history. Some guidelines for interviewing a confused older person include the following:

- Wear bright clothing to enhance the attention of the confused person.

- Go slowly and move slowly.

- Do not startle the person by approaching from the rear or by touching the person before you speak.

- Sit at the same level as the person and use a calm level tone of voice.

- Use short sentences and appropriate words.

- Call the person by the person's name.

- Keep distractions to a minimum. Turn off the radio or television and use a private room.

- Show that you are listening by nodding your head or repeating key phrases.

These techniques indicate that you are interested in what is being said and are available to the person being interviewed.

In patients with dementia or Alzheimer's disease, the functional abilities of cognition, memory, and physical capabilities that are preserved are called spared functions; those that are lost, either in whole or part, because of the disease are called impaired functions (Health Care Financing Administration *[HCFA]*, 1995). Functional abilities, both spared and impaired, should to be assessed on an ongoing basis as the disease progresses.

On the Dementia Behavior Scale (Haycox, 1984; *Table 1-5*), the higher the score, the greater is the loss of functional ability. A mental status examination, such as the Mini-Mental State *(Table 1-6)*, is used to determine the current level of cognitive function. The Mini-Mental State examination is comprehensive, can be given in 5–10 min, and has the added advantage of proven reliability and validity (Folstein, Folstein, & McHugh, 1975). Although no clinical tests specific for the diagnosis of Alzheimer's disease are currently available, a thorough clinical workup increases the accuracy of the diagnosis by ruling out other illnesses or conditions.

The following is an example of the various pictures that suggest dementing illnesses:

Mrs. Naismith was observed sitting quietly

TABLE 1-3A
Diagnostic Criteria for Dementia of the Alzheimer's Type

A. The development of multiple cognitive deficits manifested by both

    (1) memory impairment (impaired ability to learn new information or to recall previously learned information)

    (2) one (or more) of the following cognitive disturbances:

        (a) aphasia (language disturbance)

        (b) apraxia (impaired ability to carry out motor activities despite intact motor function)

        (c) agnosia (failure to recognize or identify objects despite intact sensory function)

        (d) disturbance in executive functioning (i.e., planning, organizing, sequencing, abstracting)

B. The cognitive deficits in Criteria A1 and A2 each cause significant impairment in social or occupational functioning and represent a significant decline from a previous level of functioning.

C. The course is characterized by gradual onset and continuing cognitive decline.

D. The cognitive deficits in Criteria A1 and A2 are not due to any of the following:

    (1) other central nervous system conditions that cause progressive deficits in memory and cognition (e.g., cerebrovascular disease, Parkinson's disease, Huntington's disease, subdural hematoma, normal-pressure hydrocephalus, brain tumor)

    (2) systemic conditions that are known to cause dementia (e.g., hypothyroidism, vitamin B_{12} or folic acid deficiency, niacin deficiency, hypercalcemia, neurosyphilis, HIV infection)

    (3) substance-induced conditions

E. The deficits do not occur exclusively during the course of a delirium.

F. The disturbance is not better accounted for by another Axis I disorder (e.g., Major Depressive Disorder, Schizophrenia).

Code based on type of onset and predominant features:

With Early Onset: if onset is at age 65 years or below

    290.11 With Delirium: if delirium is superimposed on the dementia

    290.12 With Delusions: if delusions are the predominant feature

    290.13 With Depressed Mood: if depressed mood (including presentations that meet full symptom criteria for a Major Depressive Episode) is the predominant feature. A separate diagnosis of Mood Disorder Due to a General Medical Condition is not given.

    290.10 Uncomplicated: if none of the above predominates in the current clinical presentation

With Late Onset: if onset is after age 65 years

    290.3 With Delirium: if delirium is superimposed on the dementia

    290.20 With Delusions: if delusions are the predominant feature

    290.21 With Depressed Mood: if depressed mood (including presentations that meet full symptom criteria for a Major Depressive Episode) is the predominant feature. A separate diagnosis of Mood Disorder Due to a General Medical Condition is not given.

    290.0 Uncomplicated: if none of the above predominates in the current clinical presentation

Specify if:

    With Behavioral Disturbance

Coding note: Also code 331.0 Alzheimer's disease on Axis III.

Reprinted with permission from *Diagnostic and statistical manual of mental disorders* (4th ed.), 1994. Washington, DC: American Psychiatric Association.

TABLE 1-3B
Diagnostic Criteria for Delirium Due to Multiple Etiologies

A. Disturbance of consciousness (i.e., reduced clarity of awareness of the environment) with reduced ability to focus, sustain, or shift attention.

B. A change in cognition (such as memory deficit disorientation, language disturbance) or the development of a perceptual disturbance that is not better accounted for by a preexisting, established, or evolving dementia.

C. The disturbance develops over a short period of time (usually hours to days) and tends to fluctuate during the course of the day.

D. There is evidence from the history, physical examination, or laboratory findings that the delirium has more than one etiology (e.g., more than one etiological general medical condition, a general medical condition plus Substance Intoxication or medication side effect).

Coding note: Use multiple codes reflecting specific delirium and specific etiologies, e.g., 293.0 Delirium Due to Viral Encephalitis: 291.0 Alcohol Withdrawal Delirium.

Reprinted with permission from *Diagnostic and statistical manual of mental disorders* (4th ed.), 1994. Washington, DC: American Psychiatric Association.

in an examination room before an interview at the memory disorder clinic. She was accompanied by her son, who was outgoing and told her story. She had a history of weight loss and had become isolated in her small apartment. In addition, she had chronic obstructive pulmonary disease and hypertension. Medications included Aldomet (methyldopa) and Tagamet (cimetidine) taken daily. Recently, she had begun to have angry outbursts toward her son when they were talking on the telephone, and she refused to accept assistance with shopping or personal care from her son or a neighbor. Her son brought her to the clinic to find out if she had the beginning of

TABLE 1-4
Basic Laboratory Tests for Causes of Possible Dementia

Test or Study	Common Problems Detected
Complete blood count	Anemia, infections
Blood chemistry	Kidney or liver disorders, diabetes
Electrolyte screen	Electrolyte imbalances
Thyroid function studies (thyroid-stimulating hormone, thyroxine, triiodothyronine, ratios)	Hypothyroidism or hyperthyroidism
Assays of vitamin B12 and folate levels	Vitamin deficiencies
VDRL tests	Syphilis
HIV tests	AIDS-related dementia

Source: Author

TABLE 1-5
The Dementia Behavior Scale

NAME_____DATE _____

TOTAL_____RATER'S INITIALS _____

LANGUAGE-CONVERSATION
0   Conversational
1   Repeats self, searches for synonyms, reticent conversation
2   Circumlocution, white lies, mild vocabulary limitation, easily led in conversation, automatisms
3   Loses thread of thought, noticeable vocabulary loss
4   Less aware of mistakes, poor syntax and sequence, perseveration, neologisms
5   Parrots words, incoherent, uncomprehending, severe vocabulary limitation
6   Mute, unresponsive

SOCIAL INTERACTION
0   Assesses, takes initiative
1   Active participant, follower
2   Bland participant, no longer empathic, loss of tact, withdrawn, clinging
3   Observer only, misidentifies close relatives, at times belligerent-defensive-suspicious
4   Out of step, poor recognition of persons, mistakes own reflection, at times menacing
5   Wanders, frequent catastrophic reaction (defiant, suspicious, combative)
6   Blank

ATTENTION AWARENESS
0   Bright, responsive
1   Requires guidance, can't recall date
2   Shortened attention, can't recall day, easily distracted
3   Wandering attention, easily tires, very few pleasures
4   Distracted by illusions, picks at imaginary lint, misidentifies objects
5   Can be engaged sporadically and briefly
6   Oblivious

SPATIAL ORIENTATION
0   Oriented
1   Orientated to immediate locus only (can't get home)
2   Hesitant, loses things
3   Disoriented to place, hides things, pack rat
4   Body disorientations, can't seat self on chair, bodily illusions, oblivious to posture
5   Hallucinating
6   Totally lost

MOTOR COORDINATION
0   Fully coordinated
1   Underactive, responsive to commands
2   Poorly coordinated, slowly moving, stumbling
3   Occasionally requires manipulation, occasionally requires assistance
4   Involuntary movements interfere, immobile, neglect of one side, requires manipulation and assistance
5   Spastic, chin on chest, wheelchair for safety, maximum physical assistance
6   Unable to ambulate, limbs contracted

BOWEL AND BLADDER
0   Self-care
1   Asks to go, needs cues to locate toilet
2   Remindable, poor hygiene occasionally, forgets to flush
3   Regular supervision, requires assistance, occasionally wet
4   Occasional fecal incontinence
5   Unpredictable, control by enema, occasional diapers
6   Fully incontinent, full-time diapers, full-time catheter

EATING AND NUTRITION
0   Self-care, weight steady, can cook
1   Needs prompting to eat, history of weight loss, burns pots
2   Needs food cut up, wanders from table, can't cook at all
3   Improper use of utensils, uses fingers, slight weight gain
4   Voraciously interested in sweets, steals food, marked weight gain, marked weight loss
5   Must be fed, eats nonfood
6   Tube fed, dysphagic

DRESS AND GROOMING
0   Appropriate self-care, well groomed
1   Won't change, poorly groomed
2   Dirty, ill-kempt, inappropriate dress, food on face
3   Misuse of clothing. misidentification of clothes, wears others' clothes, needs clothes set out
4   Dresses with instructions and help, oblivious to grooming
5   Requires full assistance
6   Must be dressed, hospital gown

Reproduced with permission from Haycox, J. A. (1984). A simple, reliable clinical behavior scale for assessing demented patients. *Journal of Clinical Psychiatry, 45*, 23–24. Copyright 1984.

TABLE 1-6
Mini-Mental Health State Exam

Patient_____ Date_____ Examiner_____

Maximum Score	Score	
		ORIENTATION
5	[ ]	What is the (year) (season) (date) (day) (month)?
5	[ ]	Where are we: (state) (county) (town) (hospital) (floor)
		REGISTRATION
3	[ ]	Name 3 objects: 1 second to say each. Then ask the patient all 3 after you have said them.
		Give 1 point for each correct answer. Then repeat them until he learns all 3. Count trials and record.
		Trials_____
		ATTENTION AND CALCULATION
5	[ ]	Serial 7's. 1 point for each correct. Stop after 5 answers. Alternatively spell "world" backwards.
		RECALL
3	[ ]	Ask for 3 objects repeated above. Give 1 point for each correct.
		LANGUAGE
9	[ ]	Name a pencil, and watch (2 points)
		Repeat the follow "No ifs, ands or buts." (1 point)
		Follow a 3-stage command: "Take a paper in your right hand, fold it in half, and put it on the floor." (3 points)
		Read and obey the following: "Close your eyes" (1 point)
_____		Write a sentence. (1 point)
TOTAL SCORE		Copy design. (1 point)

ASSESS level of consciousness along a continuum

Alert	Drowsy	Stupor	Comatose

Reprinted by permission from Folstein, M., Folstein, S., & McHugh, P. (1975). Mini-Mental State: A practical method for grading the cognitive state of patients for the clinician. *Journal of Psychiatric Research, 12*(3), 189–198. Copyright 1975.

Alzheimer's disease.

After a series of laboratory tests, a history was obtained, a physical examination was done, and arrangements were made for psychological testing. One of the psychological tests was the Beck Inventory for depression *(Table 1-7)*. The test is easily administered by the patient or by health caregiver and is reliable. Although weight loss is common in dementia and Alzheimer's disease, in Mrs. Naismith's case, the loss was attributed to clinical depression. The medications she took and her living environment contributed to the biological process of depression, which could have been mistaken for Alzheimer's disease. Furthermore, the use of cimetidine has been associated with the development of delirium (HCFA, 1995). Differentiation of delirium, depression, and dementia is vital so that vigorous approaches can be implemented.

PATHOPHYSIOLOGY

The myth that old age is invariably linked to serious intellectual and physical declines has been debunked. Aging is associated with normal biological declines in every body system, beginning with visual changes in the midtwenties. These changes may be reflected by an inability to cope with acute or chronic illnesses as a person grows older. The cumulative age-related changes influence the life of aging persons.

In general, aging occurs at the cellular level. One theory is that each cell has a genetically determined life span during which it can replicate itself a limited number of times. Structural changes in cells occur with age. In the CNS, age-related changes occur in neurons, which show signs of degeneration. As the circulation to the brain decreases, cell loss speeds up, especially in the brain. Decreases in brain weight of about 17% may occur in both men and women by the time they are 80 years old (Kaplan & Sadock, 1988).

Changes in memory and learning occur with normal biological aging. These changes do not reflect declining intelligence, but rather slowing down in the speed of learning, not the ability to learn. Simple recall declines, but verbal ability and learning skills continue.

With severe memory loss and loss of intellectual functioning, signs of degeneration of neurons are more severe. Pathological findings in Alzheimer's disease include atrophy of the cortex of the brain. Neurofibrillary tangles are found inside the neurons, and plaques are found outside the neurons. More recently recognized features of Alzheimer's disease include Hirano and Lewy bodies and granulovascular degeneration. The significance of these neuropathological changes has not been established (Burns, Howard, & Pettit, 1995).

Patients with Alzheimer's disease also have amyloid deposits in blood vessels. Research on ß-amyloid peptide, chromosomes, and other genetically related diseases, such as Down's syndrome, is being done. The exact relationship of Alzheimer's disease to ß-amyloid peptide is not known.

Changes in the structure of DNA and RNA occur in aging cells. Possible causes include genotypical programming, x-rays, noxious chemicals, and certain food products. All areas of the body are affected by aging, and no single cause of aging has been shown. Genetic factors have been implicated in some disorders that commonly occur with age, such as hypertension, coronary artery disease, and malignant neoplasms of the breast and stomach.

Determination of neurochemical deficits in Alzheimer's disease has focused on the neurotransmitters of the cholinergic system. Neurotransmitters are the chemical substances that, along with electrical impulses, relay messages or impulses from neuron to neuron in the brain and peripheral tissues. Deficits in the neurotransmitter acetylcholine were the first ones found in Alzheimer's disease. Later, deficits were discov-

TABLE 1-7
Beck Inventory

Name_____Date_____

On this questionnaire are groups of statements. Please read each group of statements carefully. Then pick out the one statement in each group which best describes the way you have been feeling the **PAST WEEK. INCLUDING TODAY!** Circle the number beside the statement you picked. If several statements in the group seem to apply equally well, circle each one. **Be sure to read all the statements in each group before making your choice.**

1.
0   I do not feel sad.
1   I feel sad.
2   I am sad all the time and I can't snap out of it.
3   I am so sad or unhappy that I can't stand it.

2.
0   I am not particularly discouraged about the future.
1   I feel discouraged about the future.
2   I feel I have nothing to look forward to.
3   I feel that the future is hopeless and that things cannot improve.

3.
0   I do not feel like a failure.
1   I feel I have failed more. than the average person.
2   As I look back on my life, all I can see is a lot of failures.
3   I feel I am a complete failure as a person.

4.
0   I get as much satisfaction out of things as I used to.
1   I don't enjoy things the way I used to.
2   I don't get real satisfaction out of anything anymore.
3   I am dissatisfied or bored with everything.

5.
0   I don't feel particularly guilty.
1   I feel guilty a good part of the time.
2   I feel quite guilty most of the time.
3   I feel guilty all of the time.

6.
0   I don't feel I am being punished.
1   I feel I may be punished.
2   I expect to be punished.
3   I feel I am being punished.

7.
0   I don't feel disappointed in myself.
1   I am disappointed in myself.
2   I am disgusted with myself.
3   I hate myself.

8.
0   I don't feel I am any worse than anybody else.
1   I am critical of myself for my weaknesses or mistakes.
2   I blame myself all the time for my faults.
3   I blame myself for everything bad that happens.

9.
0   I don't have any thoughts of killing myself.
1   I have thoughts of killing myself, but I would not carry them out.
2   I would like to kill myself.
3   I would kill myself if I had the chance.

10.
0   I don't cry any more than usual.
1   I cry more now than I used to.
2   I cry all the time now.
3   I used to be able to cry, but now I can't cry even though I want to.

11.
0   I am no more irritated now than I ever am.
1   I get annoyed or irritated more easily than I used to.
2   I feel irritated all the time now.
3   I don't get irritated at all by the things that used to irritate me.

12.
0   I have not lost interest in other people.
1   I am less interested in other people than I used to be.
2   I have lost most of my interest in other people.
3   I have lost all of my interest in other people.

13.
0   I make decisions about as well as I ever could.
1   I put off making decisions more than I used to.
2   I have greater difficulty in making decisions than before.
3   I can't make decisions at all anymore.

14.
0   I don't feel I look any worse than I used to.
1   I am worried that I am looking old or unattractive.
2   I feel that there are permanent changes in my appearance that make me look unattractive.
3   I believe that I look ugly.

15.
0   I can work about as well as before.
1   It takes an extra effort to get started at doing something.
2   I have to push myself very hard to do anything.
3   I can't do any work at all.

16.
0   I can sleep as well as usual.
1   I don't sleep as well as I used to.
2   I wake up 1–2 hours earlier than usual and find it hard to get back to sleep.
3   I wake up several hours earlier than I used to and cannot get back to sleep.

17.
0   I don't get more tired than usual.
1   I get tired more easily than I used to.
2   I get tired from doing almost anything.
3   I am too tired to do anything.

18.
0   My appetite is no worse than usual.
1   My appetite is not as good as it used to be.
2   My appetite is much worse now.
3   I have no appetite at all anymore.

19.
0   I haven't lost much weight, if any, lately.
1   I have lost more than 5 pounds.
2   I have lost more than 10 pounds.
3   I have lost more than 15 pounds.
I am purposely trying to lose weight by eating less. ☐ Yes ☐ No

20.
0   I am no more worried about my health than usual.
1   I am worried about physical problems such as aches and pains; or upset stomach; or constipation.
2   I am very worried about physical problems and it's hard to think of much else.
3   I am so worried about my physical problems that I cannot think about anything else.

21.
0   I have not noticed any recent change in my interest in sex.
1   I am less interested in sex than I used to be.
2   I am much less interested in sex now.
3   I have lost interest in sex completely.

Score: 0–9 Not Depressed, 10–15 Mild Depression, 16–23 Moderate Depression, 24–63 Severe Depression

Reproduction without author's express written consent is not permitted. Additional copies and/or permission to use this scale may be obtained from: CENTER FOR COGNITIVE THERAPY, Room 602, 133 South 36th Street, Philadelphia, PA 19104. ©1978 by Aaron T. Beck, M.D.

ered in norepinephrine, dopamine, and serotonin, either in their production or in the availability of receptor sites, where the neurotransmitter action occurs. Since the recognition of deficits in neurotransmitters in patients with Alzheimer's disease, many pharmacological treatments to add to, potentiate, or antagonize the effects of neurotransmitters have been tested (McKenry & Salerna, 1989).

More questions than answers have been raised by various theories of aging. The relationship between the biological (pathological) and the biochemical (neurochemical) changes seen in Alzheimer's disease is complex. Generally, there is more support for the idea that the neurochemical changes are due to the neuropathological changes (Burns et al, 1995). Research on genetic and physiological changes associated with Alzheimer's disease is continuing. Also, it is helpful to recognize both the normal physiological manifestations of aging and the mental changes that affect aging persons. Why one person ages so differently than others do and at such a different rate is still a great mystery.

STAGES OF DEMENTIA

The course of Alzheimer's dementia involves a gradual deterioration. Early signs and symptoms are often vague and inconclusive, this stage may last as long as 15 years. The onset of the disease is insidious and usually occurs between the ages of 50 and 80 years. Patients experience forgetfulness and personality changes, such as social withdrawal, apathy, and occasional irritable outbursts. Usually, the person is well-groomed and socially appropriate.

During the confusional stages, more severe cognitive impairments become noticeable. The early confusional stage may persist for 7 years and is characterized by the earliest recognizable deficits. Manifestations of these deficits include getting lost when driving a car, poor performance at work that is noticeable to coworkers, inability to come up with a word or name, and decreased accomplishment in demanding business and social situations. In the late confusional stage, which lasts an average of 2 years, the person has decreasing knowledge of current events and personal history, an inability to handle money, and flattening of affect (withdrawal). Denial of any cognitive problems is the affected person's major defense mechanism.

Moderate cognitive decline occurs as the early dementia phase begins. During this clinical phase, which lasts an average of 18 months, the person cannot survive without assistance. Both the ability to judge the safety of a situation and fine motor coordination are impaired. Some disorientation to time and place occurs, and the person may need help in choosing clothes, but not in eating or toileting. The person may know his or her name but not know telephone numbers or grandchildren's names.

Over a period of approximately 2 years, the manifestations of the middle phase of dementia appear. The person becomes totally dependent on the caregiver for survival and needs assistance, progressively, with all activities of daily living. Urinary and fecal incontinence begin, and emotional and personality changes increase. Often the person no longer remembers the name of his or her spouse.

Finally, in the late phase of dementia, the person becomes aphasic and inattentive. He or she cannot walk, sit up, or even hold the head up. Generalized signs of CNS involvement include quadriparesis and seizures *(Table 1-2).* The course of the disease may be 1–20 years. Generally, the younger the person is when Alzheimer's disease occurs, the more severe the disease becomes.

EXAM QUESTIONS

CHAPTER 1
QUESTIONS 1–10

1. How does the percentage of persons affected by dementia or Alzheimer's disease change after the age of 65 years?

   A. It decreases if they have no family history of the disease.

   B. It approximately doubles with each passing decade of life.

   C. It increases in those who have sedentary lifestyles.

   D. It is not affected by chronic alcoholism or AIDS.

2. Acute states of confusion accompanied by lethargy, partial consciousness, or hallucinations are best categorized as which of the following?

   A. Delirium

   B. Dementia

   C. Depression

   D. Deficiency of vitamin B or E

3. Progressive degenerative dementia is most likely to occur in which of the following conditions?

   A. Hypothyroidism

   B. Depression

   C. Creutzfeldt-Jakob disease

   D. Delirium

4. Which of the following medications would be least likely to cause depression in the elderly?

   A. Antihypertensives

   B. Sedatives

   C. Corticosteroids

   D. Nonsteroidal antiinflammatory drugs

5. What are the four *A's* of cognitive impairment?

   A. Affect, amnesia, aphasia, and apraxia

   B. Aphasia, affect, ability, and agnosia

   C. Amnesia, attitude, agnosia, and aphasia

   D. Agnosia, amnesia, apraxia, and aphasia

6. Which of the following is a normal change that occurs in the human body with aging?

   A. Neurons in the CNS do not show signs of degeneration.

   B. Brain weight decreases as much as 40% by age 80 years.

   C. Intelligence decreases markedly.

   D. Simple recall declines, but learning skills remain the same.

15

7. Which of the following statements about the early stages of Alzheimer's dementia is correct?

   A. Urinary incontinence is a major problem.

   B. The patient may not know the names of his or her spouse or grandchildren.

   C. Social withdrawal and occasional irritability are common.

   D. The person cannot survive without assistance.

8. A deficit in which of the following neurotransmitters was the first such deficit associated with Alzheimer's disease?

   A. Dopamine

   B. Adrenaline

   C. Acetylcholine

   D. Glutamate

9. The middle stage of Alzheimer's disease is characterized by which of the following?

   A. It usually lasts for 15 years.

   B. Fecal incontinence may occur.

   C. The person becomes aphasic and cannot walk or sit up.

   D. Denial is the affected person's major defense mechanism.

10. What are spared functions in patients with Alzheimer's disease?

    A. Functional abilities that are lost, in part or completely.

    B. The ability to function in a given emotional situation.

    C. Memory abilities that persist into the late stages of the disease.

    D. Cognitive, memory, and physical capabilities that are retained.

CHAPTER 2

SUPPORT FOR CAREGIVERS

CHAPTER OBJECTIVE

After completing this chapter, the reader will be able to describe the role of nurses in supporting family or staff caregivers of patients with Alzheimer's disease, how to help caregivers make choices about available types of care, and the financial and legal consequences of these decisions.

LEARNING OBJECTIVES

After studying this chapter, the reader will be able to

1. Specify three ways to manage nursing care for patients with Alzheimer's disease.

2. Recognize three stages of the caregiving career and nursing interventions for each stage.

3. Specify the correlation between feelings of the caregiver and the potential for violence.

4. Recognize interventions to aid caregivers with their feelings.

5. Distinguish the central focus of support groups for caregivers.

6. Recognize advantages and disadvantages of various levels of available care.

7. Specify the purpose of special care units for dementia.

8. Specify differences between Medicare and Medicaid.

9. Indicate the requirements of the Patient Self-Determination Act.

INTRODUCTION

As the population of the United States ages, the need to provide nursing support and increase knowledge about family caregiving grows. The Omnibus Budget Reconciliation Act of 1987 focused a nation on the long-term care needs of the elderly. Much of the emphasis since this legislation has been on providing quality care at home. The burden of this care falls on the family, who may be the primary caregiver for many years. The toll of dementia and Alzheimer's disease on caregivers has been well documented ("Clinical News," 1996; Jones & Martinson, 1992; Sayles-Cross, 1993). This chapter focuses on the role of nurses in supporting and facilitating family caregivers and on recognition of nurses in the role of the caregiver. It also discusses the family or extended family as caregivers for demented patients who live either at home or in a health care facility and how nurses can recognize common reactions to caregiving and ease the burdens. Next, it explores the importance of the environment for demented patients and compares care at home and in nursing homes. This part includes how to help families choose nursing homes, the legal and financial implications for family caregivers, and information on advanced directives and uses of Medicare and Medicaid funds.

NURSES AS CAREGIVERS

Fear, anger, and disbelief are typical reactions of family caregivers to the experience of caring for a person who has Alzheimer's disease or any other dementia. Although the names of the diseases associated with dementia may be different (see chapter 1), the nursing care, the behaviors, and the activities to be provided are essentially the same for all of them. Nurses and other health care staff members, whether at home or in a facility, may be frightened when the behavior of a demented patient is bizarre, aggressive, and hard to understand. Three keys to managing the care nurses provide in nursing homes have been suggested (Gwyther, 1985):

1. Symptom management
2. Adaptations for a therapeutic environment
3. Support for the caregivers, families, and other staff personnel.

This idea can be expanded to encompass the role of nurses as caregivers at home or in any setting where health care is provided. Managing patients' signs and symptoms and behaviors and taking steps to create a therapeutic environment are keys no matter where the demented person lives or is cared for. Most nurses encounter patients with Alzheimer's disease or another dementia in daily practice.

Supporting caregivers is a major role of professional nurses. Access to current information and the ability to convey that information to caregivers are essential. Much new information has become available, as well as a great deal of misinformation. For instance, it is known now that Alzheimer's disease is not a mental illness and that the disease is not the result of the life the person has lived. A better understanding of what is known and not known about

Alzheimer's disease can relieve fears of caregivers.

FAMILY CAREGIVERS

Researchers have looked at the reactions of caregivers and families who care for patients with dementia. One area examined is how the functional status of the demented person affects the caregiver. One study (Deimling & Bass, 1986) found that the cognitive losses of the elderly person had less effect on the health and depression of the caregiver than did the demented person's limitations in functional abilities, such as ability to perform activities of daily living. Yet, public policy and funding do not recognize the need for in-home assistance with activities of daily living unless skilled care is needed, such as after hospitalization for a major illness or injury.

Other research (Lindgren, 1993) examined the role of caregiver as a career. In this study, the role of the caregiver was conceptualized as a period in the spouse's life when the focal point is caregiving. The results showed that the active, focused role of the caregiver is similar to the role a person takes when managing his or her career. Three stages of the caregiving career were developed:

1. The encounter stage
2. The endurance stage
3. The exit stage

The career begins with the encounter stage, which involves receiving and understanding the diagnosis and adjusting to the impact of the diagnosis while learning new care skills and making changes in lifestyle. The middle stage or working stage is the endurance stage, when the heaviest workload is common as routines become established. The final stage is the exit stage, in which decisions, activities, and adjustments are made in association with the end of life.

Each stage is associated with different experiences. The encounter stage involves the grief of the caregiver for the loss of the loved one. During this phase, the need for information and the development of new skills for providing adequate personal care can be overwhelming. Educational and caregiving classes and one-to-one teaching by nurses are important.

In the endurance state, signs of both mental and physical stress are apparent as caregivers struggle through years of caregiving burdens. During this time, caregivers often have more health problems, use more prescription medications, limit social activities, take fewer vacations than before, visit less with friends, and have fewer opportunities to attend church or engage in other meaningful activities. Generally, caregivers experience a lessening of their quality of life. Finally, in the exit stage, the responsibilities of the caregiver decrease as the demented patient is admitted to a health care facility and death approaches. Looking at the needs of caregivers as a continuum of stages helps determine nursing interventions along the way.

It can also be helpful to recognize the stages of acceptance that caregivers may move through during phases of their family member's illness. Not everyone experiences all stages or in the sequence described here.

The first stage is denial, which is seen as disbelief, trying to minimize the diagnosis of Alzheimer's disease and so avoid the implications. The next stage is resistance, in which caregivers speculate that this disease will not "get" to them. Resistance is particularly apparent in caregivers who have always had good health. Next is affirmation, in which caregivers accept help and begin to discuss their feelings more openly. This stage could be the one in which a nurse helps a caregiver address difficulties in adjusting to the disease.

From affirmation, caregivers move to acceptance. During this stage, they come to terms with the illness and get on with daily life in a matter-of-fact way. Finally, growth and healing occur as a new sense of hope and determination arises. The caregiver begins to talk about the future beyond the death of the person with Alzheimer's disease. Many caregivers experience a sense of having learned and grown from their situation.

STRESS FOR CAREGIVERS

A common reaction related to caregiving (Mace & Rabins, 1991) is anger. The caregiver is angry at what has happened to him or her, angry that life has changed, angry with others who cannot or will not help, angry for being trapped in this situation, and, finally, angry at the person who is sick because of the person's irritating behavior. It is important for nurses to help family caregivers differentiate between being angry at the patient's behaviors and being angry at the patient. The behaviors can be aggravating, but they are not aimed at the caregiver personally and are part of the dementing illness.

Nurses must recognize the potential for violence in caregiving situations. A study by Pillemer and Suitor (1992) showed a strong correlation between caregivers' violent feelings and stressors such as disruptive behavior in a caregiving situation. The most important characteristic of circumstances in which actual violence occurs is being the patient's spouse and can be related to cultural norms of violence toward spouses. The exact nature and dynamics of violence in a caregiving relationship are not known. Coping with day-to-day frustrations of caregiving in ways that foster feelings of control and satisfaction (Langner, 1993) includes focusing on the present by taking one day at a time, establishing and maintaining a routine, and retelling the reasons for caregiving. The last technique encourages caregivers to sort through their feelings and continue in the role. Feelings of competence and satisfaction emerge to help sustain the caregiver.

Demands placed on caregivers involve many

recognizable areas of stress and some areas that are not as obvious. Multiple losses are experienced, such as loss of the role of spouse or child, loss of social status in the community and neighborhood, and loss of daily communication with someone who lives with the caregiver. Another demand for the caregiver is to develop and learn new roles. A husband who has never taken on housekeeping responsibilities becomes the sole caretaker of a home.

Also, families must adapt to living every day with ambiguity and uncertainty. Each day with a person with Alzheimer's disease is different, with different behaviors, and what worked yesterday may not work today. Many caregivers have never experienced the personal and interpersonal conflicts associated with caring for someone with Alzheimer's disease. Attempting to reason with someone who is unreasonable and argumentative and who behaves in a bizarre manner is disconcerting to a person who has thought that love and openness will take care of most situations.

In a survey of family caregivers by the Alzheimer's Association ("Clinical News," 1996), respondents reported spending the equivalent of two full-time jobs or an average of 69–100 hr/week caring for their loved one and dealing with the problems encountered. Four of five caregivers were women. Three quarters of respondents reported that they were occasionally depressed, and a third of those, whose family members had advanced-stage Alzheimer's disease, reported being depressed often or almost always. The majority of caregivers indicated that they and their families experienced emotional stress and depression, although the stress varied according to the phase of the illness.

Depression can be manifested as a feeling of sadness and discouragement. Distinguishing between depression, worry, grief, and helplessness is difficult *(Figure 2-1)*. Caregivers can feel apa-

thetic, listless, irritable, or anxious *(Table 2-1)*, and the feeling can last day after day and week after week (Mace, 1984). Changes in appetite and sleep can occur.

Being depressed is painful. Time spent alone in satisfying activities or in a support group may be the answer. Counseling may relieve the depression. Other times, medical help from a physician or nurse practitioner may be necessary. For some caregivers, the feelings of discouragement may go beyond the typical feelings of sadness, and antidepressant medications may be required.

Universal pitfalls of caregiving for Alzheimer's patients, which can be apparent in nursing staff as well as in family caregivers, may include the following:

- Not allowing the patient to do as much as the patient is capable of doing.
- Always putting the needs of the patient first.
- Limiting the activities of the patient by trying to protect the patient.
- Using reason or logic to assure the patient.
- Keeping expectations for the patient that are unrealistic.

Not every family caregiver, or every nurse helping a caregiver, will face the same problems. The nature and extent of the problems encountered are related to the signs and symptoms of the disease that occur, the personality of the caregiver, and the personality of the person who has Alzheimer's disease (Gwyther, 1985; Mace, 1984) The following is a list of suggestions that can make a caregiver's days easier:

1. **Stay informed.** Learn as much as possible about dementia. Behavioral management becomes more effective with more knowledge.

2. **Learn to recognize how you, as a caregiver, respond to stress.** Do you get angry or cry or withdraw or get very busy? Dealing with feel-

FIGURE 2-1
Mood Meter, What Are You Feeling?

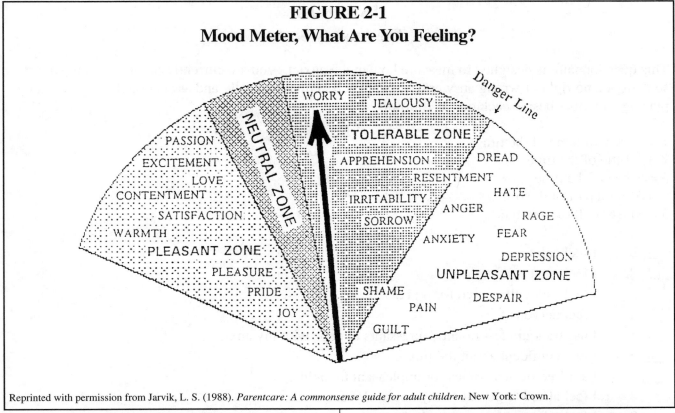

Reprinted with permission from Jarvik, L. S. (1988). *Parentcare: A commonsense guide for adult children.* New York: Crown.

ings can be stressful, but it helps to be aware of what you may do.

3. **Take care of yourself.** Develop a repertoire of activities that rejuvenate you enough to enable you to continue. Use proactive stress-reducing rituals that work for you: swimming, walking, meditating, or anything that has a calming effect on you.

4. **Recognize that other family members may have different reactions in the same circumstances.**

5. **Maintain meaningful friendships.** Help others in your support system understand the changes as the changes appear. If a person cannot overcome being negative or depressing, avoid that person.

6. **Keep the hassles small.** Decide what small daily irritant you can handle today, and ignore the rest. Practice this method and it will become easier, more like a habit.

7. **Use common sense and humor.** These are your best tools. Share your experiences with other members of your family and with other families of patients with Alzheimer's disease. In a group, what seemed so sad or frustrating may seem humorous. Let it.

SUPPORT GROUPS

Nurses must recognize that although the caregiving experience might be seen as one-dimensional, it is not all negative or positive. Nurses can help caregivers reframe or consider a different meaning for the experience. Providing education and support for caregivers and informing them about community resources are helpful (Brackley, 1992; Jacob, 1991). Involvement in a group for activities and education increases the adaptation of caregivers to their role. Group support can help caregivers find ways to get help, discover new ways of relating to their family member

TABLE 2-1
The Anxiety Scale

This questionnaire is designed to measure how much anxiety you are currently feeling. It is not a test, so there are no right or wrong answers. Answer each item as carefully and as accurately as you can by placing a number beside each one as follows:

1 = Rarely or none of the time.
2 = A little of the time.
3 = Some of the time.
4 = A good part of the time.
5 = Most or all of the time.

_____1. I feel calm.
_____2. I feel tense.
_____3. I feel suddenly scared for no reason.
_____4. I feel nervous.
_____5. I use tranquilizers or antidepressants to cope with my anxiety.
_____6. I feel confident about the future.
_____7. I am free from senseless or unpleasant thoughts.
_____8. I feel afraid to go out of my house alone.
_____9. I feel relaxed and in control of myself.
_____10. I have spells of terror or panic.
_____11. I feel afraid in open spaces or in the streets.
_____12. I feel afraid I will faint in public.
_____13. I am comfortable traveling on buses, subways, or trains.
_____14. I feel nervousness or shakiness inside.
_____15. I feel comfortable in crowds, such as shopping or at a movie.
_____16. I feel comfortable when I am left alone.
_____17. I rarely feel afraid without good reason.
_____18. Due to my fears, I unreasonably avoid certain animals, objects, or situations.
_____19. I get upset easily or feel panicky unexpectedly.
_____20. My hands, arms, or legs shake or tremble.
_____21. Due to my fears, I avoid social situations, whenever possible.
_____22. I experience sudden attacks of panic which catch me by surprise.
_____23. I feel generally anxious.
_____24. I am bothered by dizzy spells.
_____25. Due to my fears, I avoid being alone, whenever possible.

Reprinted with permission from Dr. Bruce A. Thyer, *Clinical Anxiety Scale,* University of Georgia, School of Social Work.

with dementia, and detect new ways to cope with the problems caregivers encounter.

The universality of the experience of caregiving is the central theme of support groups. Groups can be located through the Alzheimer's Association or listings in newspapers. People in support groups for families of Alzheimer's patients know what the others are going through. Grief, bizarre behavior, exhaustion, and frustration are common experiences for all types of caregivers. Blacks, Hispanics, and other minority cultures may find it more difficult to find a support group that they feel comfortable with, but all caregivers struggle with similar problems. Nurses can encourage caregivers to seek out established organizations and can assist in setting up groups in the community that meet the caregivers's special needs.

Research on caregivers has focused on what happens to both family caregivers and nursing care staff (Gwyther, 1985). Investigators have looked at the effectiveness of care techniques taught in educational and group settings. Earlier studies examined the burden on family caregivers, and now research is beginning to scrutinize the stress or burden put on professional caregivers (nurses and nursing assistants) who care for patients with Alzheimer's disease. Studies that help determine what interventions are effective for demented patients are important for nurses and will make a difference in the lives of all caregivers.

IMPORTANCE OF THE ENVIRONMENT

The influence of the environment on patients with dementia must be reevaluated on an ongoing basis. Modifications may be needed to avoid too much noise, glare, light, clutter, or verbal interactions between the patient and other people. Demented patients can be overwhelmed by changes in daily routine.

Because changes in environment are a major source of stress, caregivers may think that it is easier to care for demented patients at home (Heston & White, 1991). In a way, they are right. However, no matter how stressful hospitals, nursing homes, or day care centers may be, one or more of these facilities will almost always be necessary during the course of a dementing illness. The increase in

the severity of the demented patient's behaviors contributes to the family's decision to place the patient in a nursing facility. Behavior that may prompt placement includes combativeness, screaming, rummaging, wandering, and unmanageable incontinence. Because caring for a demented person is a 7-days-a-week, 24-hours-a-day job, alternatives should be considered before the caregiver becomes burned out and unable to continue.

ALTERNATIVES TO NURSING HOMES

Families did not always have options other than placement in a nursing home when caring for a demented patient became overwhelming. Choices do exist now, and nurses, in whatever setting families are encountered, must be able to help families make informed choices. Costs and specific needs depending on the stage of the illness are usually major concerns.

Respite care refers to various forms of home help available to families, adult day care, and short-term residential care. The providers of these services assume intermittent responsibilities for the care of the demented patient (Heston & White, 1991). Temporary help may allow a family caregiver to take a vacation or a trip or to rest up and then resume caring for the patient with renewed enthusiasm. Respite care is often provided by non-professionals who have special training in dealing with demented persons or through a local Alzheimer's Association.

Respite care can be given in adult day care centers designed specifically for confused persons. Families can avail themselves of the services daily or several times a week. The emphasis is on keeping the demented individual active as long as possible. Daily fees are $15 to $80. Nurses can assist family caregivers by becoming informed about local day care services, including if the services center their programs on patients in one stage or another of Alzheimer's disease. If wandering is a problem, special programs should be in place to curb the behavior. Low staff-to-patient ratios and active, stimulating but calm environments should be provided.

Respite care at home can be arranged through health care agencies or other community-based agencies. Another in-home service is the provision of equipment, such as wheelchairs and walkers, by community and fraternal groups. Transportation and Meals on Wheels are available to provide services at home. Nurses should be aware that most respite care is provided by nonprofessionals. Therefore, if a patient with Alzheimer's disease has complex needs, respite care in the home may not be advisable; home health care may be needed instead. Some organizations have financial support for families who need this type of in-home support.

Nursing homes, hospitals, and other care facilities can offer respite care for several days or weeks in an emergency or during a vacation by the caregiver. Nurses should be informed about local nursing homes and residential care facilities that offer respite care. Nurses should also be familiar with both federal and state regulations on respite care, because each state may enact its own regulations and laws. An added benefit of residential respite care for patients in the advanced stages of Alzheimer's disease is that their caregivers may then realize that it is time to arrange for long-term care in a nursing home.

Foster care homes, board and care homes, and assisted living facilities or adult congregate living facilities are another option for families of patients with Alzheimer's disease. When a less restrictive and less intensive form of care is needed and a mix of services is required, these programs provide choices (HCFA, 1991). Nurses should know if state regulations govern the type and extent of services that can be offered.

Facilities offer assisted living for patients with a wide variety of needs. In most facilities of this type, the patient or family pays a flat rate for certain contracted services, meals, and so forth. Any additional services are paid for as needed. Nurses should be aware of what is available in their area of the country. They should find out if the services a facility advertises or promises families of patients with Alzheimer's disease can be legally offered and are provided by the facility. Families should avoid facilities that charge exorbitant prices merely to "lock up" demented patients in a unit with few or no programs to retain the functional abilities the patients still have.

Many facilities are developing special programs for demented patients. Currently, little or no public funding is available for the assisted living level of care, so families often assume the financial burden. As advocates, nurses can ask questions about programming and use their eyes and ears in the community to verify what is being advertised about facilities of this type. When they encounter someone who has used a service or visits regularly, they can get that person's opinion and recommendation. Nurses are in a unique position to learn about community resources and become an authority on their community. When a patient with Alzheimer's disease needs 24-hour nursing care and supervision, a nursing home may be the best or only answer.

CHOOSING A NURSING HOME

Forty to forty-five percent of everyone who became 65 years old in 1990 will stay in a nursing home at least once in their lifetime (HCFA, 1991). At least half of those admitted to nursing homes will have some type of dementing illness such as Alzheimer's disease. Many times the choice of a nursing home is made in a crisis. Nurses can help caregivers and patients with

Alzheimer's consider the options in advance. The Caregiver Checklist *(Table 2-2)* is a system to help caregivers look at future needs. Caregivers may never need a nursing home, but the problems of trying to locate a good nursing home quickly are monumental. Families can end up losing money or using facilities they do not like because they did not anticipate the need.

If a caregiver has time (the patient with Alzheimer's disease is not hospitalized or does not need immediate placement), he or she can talk to the local Alzheimer's Association and ask friends or relatives for suggestions. Another source of information on good nursing homes is the local library, ombudsman, or nursing home advocacy group. Federal law requires the disclosure of information about nursing homes that have not met minimum standards.

Caregivers must be sure, however, that survey results available in the library reflect the current condition of local nursing homes. In the 1980s, studies recognized problems with the quality of life in many nursing homes in the United States. Consequently, nursing home reforms went into effect in 1990 that are designed to enhance both the quality of care and the quality of life for residents in nursing homes.

Seeking referrals can help caregivers avoid frustration and focus their search. As the search continues, caregivers can make telephone calls, which can eliminate some facilities. The following are key questions to ask (HCFA, 1991):

1. Is the nursing home certified to participate in Medicare and Medicaid programs?

2. What are the facility's admission requirements for residents?

3. What is the typical resident in the facility like? (If the caregiver requires a special program for a patient with Alzheimer's disease, and the facility specializes in subacute care, the facility might not be a good choice.)

4. Does the nursing home require signing over of personal property or real estate in exchange for care?

5. Does the facility have a waiting list, or does it have vacancies?

The location of a nursing home is another consideration. Many elderly caregivers prefer not to drive at night, so having their family member in a facility near their own home is important to them. Caregivers should visit several nursing homes, ideally more than once. At least one visit to each home should be made in the late morning or at noontime so they can observe whether residents are out of bed and whether a meal is being served. Preparing and serving meals are two of the most important functions provided by nursing home staff.

Caregivers should take the time to observe serving of a meal. They should look at how residents are assisted with eating, how special adaptive equipment is used, and how much time is allowed for residents to eat. For patients with Alzheimer's disease, cueing and suggestions by staff for recalling lost abilities such as how to use utensils are important. Caregivers should ask to sample the food and should observe whether residents appear to be enjoying the meal.

If the residents of a nursing home are in physical restraints, representatives of the facility should be asked about the home's philosophy of using restraints and about what activities and rehabilitation are available to keep residents free from restraints. The use of both physical and chemical restraints is strictly limited by federal regulations. A restraint cannot be used because of lack of staff and must be ordered by a physician. When a medication is used, staff personnel must monitor the behaviors that justified the use of the chemical restraint and must make a record of any side effects.

While visiting nursing homes, caregivers should talk to residents and staff members.

TABLE 2-2
Caregiver Checklist

The following checklist will assist the caregiver.
MEDICAL:
____ Obtain a complete medical examination from a physician
____ Proper diagnosis—possible second opinion
____ Consultation with physician about what to expect
____ Evaluation in terms of level of functioning
____ Identify medication currently taken; obtain full medical history

LEGAL: Contact an attorney for advice regarding:
____ Power of Attorney (in/out of state)
____ Will
____ Living Will—Passed as legal enactment by Florida Legislature in Spring 1984
____ Guardianship
____ Any other possible concerns

FINANCIAL: Determine if person can manage financial matters. If not, someone should take responsibility of:
____ Checking account (bill payments)
____ Savings account
____ Other assets (stocks, bonds, CDs)
____ Real estate or other property owned
____ Locate and review all insurance policies (medical, life, disability, VA, car, house, etc.)
____ Locate safety deposit keys and signature authorizations (also personal safe combinations)
____ Check for Waiver of Premium clause on insurance policies
____ Identify monthly income sources (Social Security, direct deposits, pension, etc.)
____ Regarding Social Security, do you want to be made Representative Payee?
____ Has Social Security been applied for?

FUNERAL/BURIAL ARRANGEMENTS:
____ Does the person prefer burial or cremation?
____ Have arrangements been made for purchase of burial lot, casket, funeral, etc.?
____ Autopsy arrangements
____ Religious/spiritual preference

CAREGIVING:
____ Contact the local AGE LINK for pertinent information
____ Obtain knowledge of community resources by contacting Helpline
____ Develop a plan for care—include several alternatives
____ Utilize available programs such as Adult Day Care, Respite, Volunteers, etc.
____ Perform a safety sweep throughout the home

OTHER:
____ Driving (You must judge when the person can no longer operate a motor vehicle safely)
____ I.D. bracelet for the person, in case of wandering

Adapted with permission from *Caregivers Check List,* Alzheimer's Association, Fort Myers, FL.

Questions to ask include what the residents and staff members like about their home, what they would change if they could, and what they do if they do not like something and whom they talk to. The answers can provide a valuable insight into the quality of life in the home. *Table 2-3* lists common concerns about the care of nursing home residents with dementia. After touring various homes, talking to residents and staff, and observing the conditions of the home, caregivers can form their own impression. Trusting their own instincts and perceptions is necessary.

SPECIAL CARE UNITS FOR PATIENTS WITH DEMENTIA

Before a patient with Alzheimer's disease is admitted to a nursing home, it is essential to inquire about the environment and systems in place in the nursing home to support demented patients. Most nursing homes integrate confused residents with alert and oriented, frail elderly residents (Buckwalter, 1993). Staff personnel may be uninformed about the special needs of patients with Alzheimer's disease and other dementias. Confrontations between demented patients and other residents, staff members, and family can lead to the tendency to use physical and chemical restraints for safety and peace.

So-called special care units have been developed to address the care issues of demented persons. Most units have approximately 20 residents in single- and double-occupancy rooms. At least five characteristics make dementia units special:

1. Staff selection and training
2. Activity programs developed for demented patients
3. Programs for the families of demented patients
4. Environmental alterations, including decor

5. Admission criteria that specify patients must have Alzheimer's disease or some other dementia.

Currently, there is no definition of a special care unit and no information on the best staff training or staffing patterns. Activities for the residents and programs for their families vary greatly, as do admission criteria based on treatment philosophy. The underlying purpose of these units is to maintain or increase the functional status of the demented patients. Much of the research supports the notion that segregating demented patients from the rest of the residents leads to a better quality of life. However, more studies are needed on what makes a dementia unit special. Caregivers should ask questions about the programs and environment of any unit dedicated to patients with Alzheimer's disease and find out what makes the unit special.

FINANCIAL AND LEGAL IMPLICATIONS

Caregivers make tremendous financial sacrifices to care for patients with Alzheimer's disease ("Clinical News," 1996). As dedicated and determined as most caregivers are, the burden is often too much to bear alone. Help for caregivers is fragmented, not always available, and sometimes expensive. For most caregivers, finding ways to finance nursing home care is a major concern. Four basic methods are used:

1. **Personal resources:** About one-half of nursing home residents pay for their care from their own resources. When their resources are depleted, they apply for Medicaid.

2. **Private insurance:** Purchasing long-term care insurance is another option. If this option is being considered, caregivers should check the length of time that preexisting conditions are excluded and, of course, whether the insurance

has any permanent exclusions for Alzheimer's disease.

3. **Medicaid**

4. **Medicare**

Medicare and Medicaid, the major government reimbursement programs for the care of older persons, spend most of their dollars on nursing homes and hospitals. Much less of Medicare spending goes to cover in-home costs of care. Medicare is designed to cover acute care, not long-term care (Mace & Rabins, 1991).

Medicare may pay for at least part of nursing home costs for up to 100 days per benefit period for patients who require intensive rehabilitation or skilled nursing care *(HCFA,* 1991). Patients with Alzheimer's disease or dementia usually do not warrant this type of care. However, if a patient with Alzheimer's disease or dementia has an acute illness or injury that does require these services, Medicare may cover the cost of the services. Nursing homes must work closely with discharge planners to avoid problems and be sure that only persons requiring skilled services are admitted to skilled parts of nursing homes. A convenient appeal process is available to residents in nursing homes who think they have been wrongly denied Medicare benefits.

Qualifying for Medicaid benefits can be frustrating and complicated, but Medicaid can pay for nursing facility care when more than room and board but not skilled care is required. The patient must meet income and resource eligibility guidelines. Financial criteria vary from state to state, so nurses should help caregivers contact the local state Medicaid agency as early as possible. Recent changes in Medicaid law related to "spousal impoverishment" provisions protect a certain amount of income and resources for a spousal caregiver still living at home when the partner needs nursing home care.

Community agencies can lessen the financial burden on caregivers. Caregivers can contact the local area agency on aging (listed in the telephone book) or the state department of elder affairs or aging. These agencies can refer callers to community resources or to the information hot lines of local age-related services. The Alzheimer's Association and local churches are other sources for community support services.

Financial advice can be obtained from financial planners, accountants, and tax professionals so that caregivers make prudent decisions about money management. All agree that caregivers should consult an attorney about legal strategies before nursing home care is needed for a patient with Alzheimer's disease. Discussions should include legal arrangements, such as joint checking and savings accounts, power of attorney agreements, and guardianships or trusts.

When the Patient Self-Determination Act went into effect in 1991, it ensured that individuals have the final say about how much and what kind of medical treatment they receive (MacKay, 1992). Most states now require that health care facilities ask each patient if the patient has an advanced directive and must record the patient's response. Additionally, facilities and agencies must educate their staff, patients, and the public about having and implementing advanced directives. Simply having an advanced directive is not sufficient to ensure that the individual's wishes will be respected.

Laws on drawing up and implementing living wills vary from state to state. Nurses should familiarize themselves with state laws in their practice state. In general, a living will outlines a person's wishes for sustaining and maintaining medical treatments and nutrition in the future. For persons who become demented, the living will assists the designated health care surrogate or proxy to make decisions based on the demented person's wishes. Many persons, for instance, have voiced specific desires about the use of feeding tubes or cardiopul-

---

TABLE 2-3

Frequently Cited Complaints and Concerns About the Care Providers for Nursing Home Residents With Dementia

- Dementia in nursing home residents often is not carefully or accurately diagnosed and sometimes is not diagnosed at all.

- Acute and chronic illnesses, depression. and sensory impairments that can exacerbate cognitive impairment in an individual with dementia frequently are not diagnosed or treated.

- There is a pervasive sense of nihilism about nursing home residents with dementia; that is, a general feeling among nursing home administrators and staff that nothing can be done for these residents.

- Nursing home staff members frequently are not knowledgeable about dementia or effective methods of caring for residents with dementia. They generally are not aware of effective methods of responding to behavioral symptoms in residents with dementia.

- Psychotropic medications are used inappropriately for residents with dementia, particularly to control behavioral symptoms.

- Physical restraints are used inappropriately for residents with dementia, particularly to control behavioral symptoms.

- The basic needs of residents with dementia, e.g., hunger, thirst, and pain relief, sometimes are not met because the individuals cannot identify or communicate their needs, and nursing home staff members may not anticipate the needs.

- The level of stimulation and noise in many nursing homes is confusing for residents with dementia. Nursing homes generally do not provide activities that are appropriate for residents with dementia.

- Nursing homes generally do not provide enough exercise and physical movement to meet the needs of residents with dementia.

- Nursing homes do not provide enough continuity in staff and daily routines to meet the needs of residents with dementia.

- Nursing home staff members do not have enough time or flexibility to respond to the individual needs of residents with dementia.

- Nursing home staff members encourage dependency in residents with dementia by performing personal care functions, such as bathing and dressing, for them instead of allowing and assisting the residents to perform these functions themselves.

- The physical environment of most nursing homes is too "institutional" and not "home-like" enough for residents with dementia.

- Most nursing homes do not provide cues to help residents find their way.

- Most nursing homes do not provide appropriate space for residents to wander.

- Most nursing homes do not make use of design features that could support residents' independent functioning.

- The needs of families of residents with dementia are not met in many nursing homes.

Adapted from Health Care Financing Administration. (1995). *Surveyor's guidebook on dementia* (Pub. No. 386-897/33457). Washington, DC: U.S. Government Printing Office.

monary resuscitation.

By planning ahead, patients with Alzheimer's disease can discuss their wants and desires with their caregivers, and the caregivers can assist an attorney in preparing a durable power of attorney for health care. Many states have preprinted forms that are easy to use and readily available. Caregivers should not use a standard power of attorney form, because this form is only for managing property, not for making decisions about health care.

As the dementia progresses, the designated person can make all the health care decisions in collaboration with health care providers. When a person with Alzheimer's disease is dying, the decisions of the designated person, based on knowledge of the demented patient's wishes, take legal precedence over the decisions of others involved with the patient. Families sometimes find it difficult to face these decisions. Nurses occupy a unique place in offering guidance and support to family caregivers and to patients with Alzheimer's disease. They can encourage caregivers and patients to discuss these issues and plan ahead.

Attorneys and the Alzheimer's Association can help demented patients and their families plan for the eventuality of needing someone to act in the demented patient's best interests. Some states specify by law which close relatives can make medical decisions without a guardianship. If needed, a petition may be filed with the court to request a guardian of the person with dementia. Making formal arrangements can prevent serious headaches for families when disputes or conflicts occur.

SUMMARY

Planning ahead is the best way to avoid some of the stresses of caregiving for patients with Alzheimer's disease. Nurses offer services through out the community to assist and support family caregivers in taking care of not only the patients but also the caregivers themselves. The concerns of family caregivers correlate with the problems encountered by nursing staff caregivers. Research is determining strategies for managing stress of the caregivers and techniques for successfully managing the behavioral issues of demented patients. Making choices about the available continuum of care is complicated, and nurses should be informed about the choices caregivers make as the caregivers maneuver through the financial and legal network surrounding the decisions that are made.

EXAM QUESTIONS

CHAPTER 2
Questions 11–20

11. Nurses can help caregivers manage patients with Alzheimer's disease by doing which of the following?

    A. Teaching strategies to control signs and symptoms

    B. Looking for cues in the environment

    C. Accessing financial providers

    D. Recognizing that caregivers must function independently

12. Which of the following nursing interventions would be most helpful during the encounter stage of the caregiving career?

    A. Providing education on caregiving

    B. Determining how the caregiver reacts to stress

    C. Finding respite care in a residential facility

    D. Assisting with grieving

13. What is the single most important characteristic of situations in which violence may occur in caregiving?

    A. A daughter or son is the caregiver.

    B. Attempts are made to reason with a demented patient.

    C. The patient has a loss of functional ability.

    D. The spouse is the caregiver.

14. Which of the following is a technique that helps caregivers learn how to cope with their feelings?

    A. Recognizing that in a difficult situation others around them will see things the same as they do

    B. Going for a walk every morning

    C. Putting the needs of the person with Alzheimer's disease first

    D. Learning as much as they can about Alzheimer's disease

15. Support groups help caregivers of patients with Alzheimer's disease focus on which of the following?

    A. How unique each person is

    B. Common experiences that every caregiver encounters

    C. How to limit the activities of the person with Alzheimer's disease

    D. How to explain things to a person who has Alzheimer's disease

16. What is one benefit of adult day care for caregivers?

    A. Programs are available for patients with specific behavioral problems.

    B. Public funding is easily arranged.

    C. The emphasis is on providing rest so the person can be more active at home.

    D. The staff-to-patient ratio is 1:1.

17. Which of the following is an advantage that respite care provides to the caregiver of a patient with Alzheimer's disease?

    A. Care is provided in the home by well-trained professionals.

    B. When provided in the home, it is useful when the patient has complex care needs.

    C. Care can be provided in adult day care centers.

    D. When provided in a residential facility, it cannot exceed 24 hours.

18. What is the chief purpose of special care units for demented patients?

    A. To train staff personnel to care for demented patients

    B. To increase the facility's revenues

    C. To maintain the functional abilities of patients who have dementia

    D. To involve the patients' families in special programs

19. Which of the following statements about Medicare and Medicaid is correct?

    A. Medicare is not designed to handle acute care needs.

    B. Residents in nursing homes can appeal decisions about Medicare payments for services.

    C. Medicaid eligibility criteria are established by the federal government.

    D. The spouse of the person attempting to qualify for Medicaid must spend all remaining money before Medicaid funds will be provided.

20. The Patient Self-Determination Act requires which of the following?

    A. All terminally ill patients must have advanced directives.

    B. Health care facilities must educate staff members and patients about advanced directives.

    C. Health care agencies and facilities must implement each patient's living will.

    D. Spouses must be allowed to make decisions for patients with Alzheimer's disease.

CHAPTER 3

THERAPEUTIC APPROACHES

CHAPTER OBJECTIVE

After completing this chapter, the reader will be able to recognize common therapeutic approaches for managing the behavior of demented patients and how to incorporate the approaches into nursing practice.

LEARNING OBJECTIVES

After studying this chapter, the reader will be able to

1. Recognize factors that prompted the development of various therapeutic approaches for managing the behavior of demented patients.

2. Differentiate benefits of the therapeutic approaches of reality orientation, reminiscence, validation therapy, and humor therapy.

3. Indicate various techniques used in reality orientation, reminiscence, validation therapy, and humor therapy.

4. Specify which therapeutic approaches are best for patients in early and late stages of Alzheimer's disease.

5. Indicate characteristics of humor therapy.

6. Recognize factors in the nursing home environment that influence the lives of patients with dementia.

7. Recognize factors to be considered in the nursing assessment of the psychosocial environment of patients with dementia.

8. Specify aspects of the organizational environment of an agency or facility.

INTRODUCTION

A loving person lives in a loving world.

A hostile person lives in a hostile world:

Everyone you meet is your mirror.

Ken Keyes, Jr.

Caring for someone with Alzheimer's disease poses many challenges for both nurses and nonprofessional caregivers. Bizarre behaviors and memory problems make it difficult to understand and work with impaired patients. The things patients do, their behaviors, can be the most distressing part of dementia or Alzheimer's disease. This chapter discusses therapeutic approaches to dealing with common problems.

One way to approach irritating and bizarre behaviors is to attempt to understand what they mean. In other words, why do people act the way they do? We know that dementia and Alzheimer's disease damage the brain so that the patient cannot make sense out of what he or she sees and hears. Memory loss, anger, agitation, and other behaviors can cause embarrassment, frustration, and exhaustion to those providing care. Exploring what works best for each caregiver and what has worked for others helps.

The philosophy of any organization or person is what guides the practice and sets the priorities of that organization or person. The philosophy of nurses who must cope with a patient with dementia most likely will represent a person-centered, individualized approach (Rader, 1996a). Health care facilities may have a philosophy statement, but if the statement cannot be translated into action, it will not be helpful for the nurses who work there.

REALITY ORIENTATION

The basic format of reality orientation includes reminding patients with dementia or Alzheimer's disease who they are and who is speaking to them, providing information about time and place, and giving a description about what is going on (Moffat, 1994). It is important for caregivers to speak clearly, keeping statements brief and specific. Demented patients are encouraged to rehearse the information given and to talk with staff members and with others, if in a group. The original goal of reality orientation was to meet the sensory and emotional needs of patients who required long-term care. The needs would be met by (1) promoting one-to-one personal contacts in which nursing assistants would spend more time with residents, (2) providing stimulating activities for residents, and (3) encouraging certain attitudes in staff personnel.

The guidelines can be summarized as follows (Moffat, 1994):

1. New information is presented in a variety of formats, including routine communication and special learning groups.

2. Incorrect or confused behavior or actions are corrected by staff.

3. Prompting, rehearsal, and reinforcement of adaptive behavior are used.

4. Memory aides, such as reality orientation boards with date and time, are used to alleviate memory problems.

Reality orientation has been modified over time to a more acceptable approach in which the aim is for staff members to respond to residents' initiatives rather than to initiate the interactions. An alternative to verbal information is to teach demented patients to follow appropriately posted signs to find their own way around in the facility environment or at home. Using external memory aides such as appointment books, alarm watches, and daily routine schedules may maintain memory in patients in the early stages of Alzheimer's disease.

Historically, reality orientation was the mainstay of therapeutic activities in nursing homes, and it is a requirement in some states for long-term-care licensing (Ebersole & Hess, 1994). The blanket application of reality orientation procedures is questioned by many. It seems cruel and unnecessary to say to a confused patient, Your mother has been dead for 20 years, and you are now living in Sunnybrook Nursing Home. Other more humane and realistic ways can be used to communicate with patients who have dementia. At times, reality orientation is a useful tool to orient a demented person to reality, especially during the early stages of the disease.

Reality orientation should be used with discrimination. Attitudes of staff members are significant when implementing reality orientation. Active friendliness and a matter-of-fact approach are supportive and build self-esteem. The first determination for a demented patient should be whether relating to the external world or surroundings is of more importance than joining the patient in his or her time and place. In a clinical setting, an emphasis on reality orientation can lead to increased agitation and anxiety. Patients with dementia may become too impaired to benefit from memory training such as reality orientation (Wilson & Moffat, 1994).

REMINISCENCE

Reminiscing is considered a particularly adaptive function during the last stage of life. Life review was introduced by Butler in 1963 as a way to review the past in an attempt to examine conflicts and resolve and reconcile them or make order and meaning from them. The concept of reminiscing has been used in many settings and for many purposes. Apparently, patients with dementia or Alzheimer's disease often retain remote memories long after more short-term memory is gone. The retention of remote memory can be used by nurses to maintain patients' sense of self-esteem and identity (Ebersole & Hess, 1994). Because old memories are not judged for accuracy, they do not threaten the adequacy of the person who is reminiscing.

During group reminiscing, triggers or aids can be used to access the memories. Such aids include music, photographs, foods, and smells that initiate recall and discussion of memories (Burns et al, 1995). The value of group reminiscing lies in the enjoyment and satisfaction it gives to patients, and to their families, if the families are involved. Although reminiscence therapy has not had significant effects on cognition or behavior, it has helped relieve depression among persons with dementia.

Guidelines for nurses for reminiscence therapy include the following:

- When beginning, discuss with the patients the normal characteristics of a life review.

- Give each patient the chance to recap events in his or her life. Ask questions such as "What do you remember about your first day of school?" or make requests such as "Tell us about the first doll you had."

- Help patients put their lives in a broader or a different perspective. For instance, ask them, "How did you manage?" or "Who helped you get through that?" or "How would you change that now?"

- Make connections between past hopes and dreams and the future, or make connections between members of the group to show common bonds.

- Focus on the individual as the central person in any story told. For example, ask, "What were you doing then?"

- Work toward the goal of increasing self-esteem of each person by recognizing the person's individuality.

- Share some of your own memories as long as it helps the demented person share his or her memories.

Reminiscing has many therapeutic values. It can make memories more acceptable as they are discussed in the group and can enrich the daily lives of persons who can experience life fully. Sharing of memories by group members can stimulate other memories, and talking about the loss of pets can help members recognize their coping styles for grief and loss. Other benefits include healing loneliness and isolation, giving a sense of continuity to life, and providing understanding from one generation to another (Rader, 1996a).

Studies have shown that reminiscing can lead to positive changes in the attitude of nursing assistants toward elderly persons in a nursing home (Pictrowicz & Johnson, 1991). In addition, reminiscing requires little additional effort or time, so it does not intrude on the staff's work tasks. Another possible benefit is that nursing assistants may perceive elderly residents as more vital and unique, and this perception may increase the assistants' own self-esteem as health care workers whose work has often been undervalued or devalued.

The patients who reminisce most effectively

are those who are also highly functional. Reminiscence should be part of a comprehensive program to address the emotional and cognitive and behavioral needs of patients who have dementia or Alzheimer's disease. The loss of verbal ability and intact memory in the middle and later stages of Alzheimer's disease makes reminiscence therapy less appropriate for patients in these stages.

VALIDATION THERAPY

Validation means accepting patients with Alzheimer's disease who return to the past to survive present-day losses. It tunes into patients' inner world and helps them restore the past by reliving good times and resolving past conflicts. Based on respect and empathy, validation helps reduce stress, enhance dignity, and increase happiness (Feil, 1982).

The foundation of validation therapy is to examine the meaning of apparently senseless or bizarre behavior rather than focus on the reality of the situation. For example, if an old woman in a nursing home says there was a man under her bed last night, it does not help to argue with her. But caregivers cannot agree with her either, because on some level, she knows the man was not there even though she saw him clearly in her mind's eye. What they can do is rephrase what she said, "You saw a man in here? Who was he? When did you see him? What did he look like?" If a caregiver can get the woman to talk about the woman's feelings and validate that they are real, they lose their strength. If they are ignored, they only become stronger.

Validating a patient's particular need or feeling can restore self-esteem and promote a deeper understanding of the patient by staff members. Validation therapy involves following the patient's lead and responding to the issues that are important to the patient rather than interrupting to supply factual data, as in reality orientation. Even the most

weird or fantastic words or actions carry a message if caregivers are willing to listen. It does not mean that the patient's inappropriate words or actions are reinforced. Nurses should respond sensitively and reorient the patient only when they have a legitimate reason for doing so.

Consider this example: Mrs. Smythe continually stuffs paper tissues in her purse. The nurse asks if the paper is important. When Mrs. Smythe nods yes, the nurse suggests that being organized and putting things where they belong is important. The nurse asks if stuffing the tissues away makes Mrs. Smythe feel better. When Mrs. Smythe responds affirmatively, the nurse has validated the action and its meaning to Mrs. Smythe. Making sense of the activity is helped by the nurse's knowledge that Mrs. Smythe was a bookkeeper and often put important papers in envelopes and file cabinets. Pointing out that Mrs. Smythe no longer has a job and lives in Sunnybrook Nursing Home now would serve no useful purpose. However, one approach, in this instance, could be to occupy Mrs. Smythe in stuffing envelopes as a purposeful and useful activity.

Techniques used by health care providers during validation therapy include the following:

*   Use nonthreatening and factual words to build trust.

*   Ask questions such as who, what, when, where, and how, but not why.

*   Validate feelings only after they are expressed.

*   Rephrase the statement, but be somewhat vague. Repeat in your own words what was said; use the same pitch, tempo, and even facial expression as those used by the patient.

*   Use polarity. Ask the patient to describe the extreme form of his or her experience. Try to help the patient imagine the opposite. Was there a time when the behavior, or whatever, did not occur?

- Reminisce. Explore the past to establish trust and find familiar coping methods to use again.

- For patients who are less verbal, use touch, voice, and eye contact. Music helps.

Validation therapy is useful in restoring a sense of well-being in nursing home populations that include patients with Alzheimer's disease (Feil, 1987). It can increase trust, improve speech, increase clearness of thinking, and provide more social interaction. Validation therapy is a patient-centered therapy rooted in the tradition of transactional and Jungian analyses (Burns et al, 1995). Although some medical practitioners are skeptical about the scientific rationale for its use, those who have seen the beneficial results continue to advocate for its use.

HUMOR THERAPY

Laughter is like changing a baby's diaper; it doesn't permanently solve any problems, but it makes things more acceptable for a while.

Ashleigh Brilliant

The medical and educational world has been intolerant of humor. According to one story, a nurse educator was walking down the hallway one day, outside a classroom full of nursing students. The students burst out laughing and continued laughing for several minutes. The instructor commented to another much younger nursing instructor, "There can't be anything productive going on in there; listen to them laugh." Yet, health care and education's attitude toward humor has another side, an openness and flexibility that has been recognized since ancient times.

Probably the most dramatic and well-documented event in recent history that brought humor into the spotlight for health care was the illness of Norman Cousins (Dossey, 1996). In 1964, after the diagnosis of a crippling and painful disease, anky-losing spondylitis with severe inflammation of the spine and joints, Cousins checked out of the hospital and into a hotel. He had learned about the possible relationship between psychological stress and certain diseases. He spent the time in the hotel watching Laurel and Hardy films, the Marx Brothers, and clips from *Candid Camera,* the television show. In 1989, in his book, *Head First: The Biology of Hope,* Cousins speculated on how he literally laughed himself back to health. A new specialty, humor therapy, was born.

Patty Wooten (1996), a critical care nurse and founder of Jest for the Health of It Services, has done research on the role of humor in helping nurses develop a greater sense of control to overcome professional burnout. After a 6-hr humor training course, she found, "If one is encouraged and guided to use humor, one can gain a sense of control in your life." Staying in touch with the playful, childlike nature within themselves is more difficult for nurses because of the seriousness of their work. Caring for patients with Alzheimer's disease is often stressful. Feeling out of control is a natural tendency. Many times nurses cannot control the situations presented to them, but they can always control their reaction to the situation (Laurenhue, 1996).

One of the goals of humor therapy for nurses is to try to understand where the other person is coming from. First, nurses must understand themselves and become aware of the choices they make every day. This is the first step in taking responsibility for themselves. Being conscious of what they are doing brings persons' values and actions into congruence *(Table 3-1).* Developing a sense of humor is easier when persons feel good about themselves.

The most important part of understanding another person's perspective is to realize that all behavior has meaning. Nurses can use their sense of humor to add enjoyment to the day of patients who have Alzheimer's disease. With demented

TABLE 3-1
50 Excuses for a Closed Mind

1. We tried that before	26. Where'd you dig that one up?
2. Our place is different	27. We did all right without it
3. It costs too much	28. It's never been tried before
4. That's not my job	29. Let's shelve it for the time being
5. It's too radical a change	30. Let's form a committee
6. They're too busy to do that	31. I don't see the connection
7. We don't have the time	32. It won't work in our area
8. Not enough help	33. The board would never go for it
9. The staff will never buy it	34. Let's all sleep on it
10. It's against facility policy	35. It can't be done
11. The union will scream	36. It's too much trouble to change
12. Runs up our overhead	37. It won't pay for itself
13. We don't have the authority	38. I know a person who tried it
14. Let's get back to reality	39. It's impossible
15. That's not our problem	40. We've always done it this way
16. I don't like the idea	41. The administrators won't buy it
17. You're right, but...	42. We'd lose money in the long run
18. You're two years ahead of your time	43. Don't rock the boat
19. We're not ready for that	44. That's what we can expect from the staff
20. It isn't in the budget	45. Has anyone else ever tried it?
21. Can't teach an old dog new tricks	46. Let's look into it further
22. Good thought, but impractical	47. Quit dreaming
23. Let's give it more thought	48. That won't work in our facility
24. We'll be the laughing stock	49. That's too ivory tower
25. Not that again	50. It's too much work

Adapted with permission from Larenhue, K. (1996). *Caregiving with humor and creativity.*

patients, body language and tone of voice carry more credibility than words do.

Suggestions on how to get in the humor habit include the following:

- Turn off the television and be sociable. People laugh 30 times more often in a social setting than they do when alone.

- Learn something new. Try an activity, such as in-line skating, that you may not excel at, and try it with someone you like.

- Choose your friends carefully. A friend you laugh with is a treasure. Unload the duds, and cultivate the gems.

- Do not be lazy. It is not a bother to make the extra effort to be silly or funny. Make wisecracks or use puns.

- Cultivate running jokes. When you find yourself in a moment of shared hilarity, make the most of it. Repeat it, and keep laughing.

- Master the art of comic complaining. Exaggerate and overstate. Poke fun at yourself.

- Share the joke. When you hear or read something funny, pass it along and laugh all over again.

- Get a pet. Stupid pet tricks launched David Letterman's career. Cats and dogs crack people up. And you do not have to train pets to be funny.

- Start the day with a laugh. Fifteen minutes of cartoons such as the Roadrunner can set the silliness mood for the rest of the day.

Preschoolers laugh an average of 400 times per day. Adults laugh an average of 15 times per day. Many nurses are their own worst enemies, constantly ridiculing themselves for real or imagined mistakes as they enter a "serious" profession such as nursing. Studies have shown that most people say four times as many bad things as good things about themselves. People who are in control can control their reactions to behavior that is bizarre or not easily understood, even when the situation cannot be controlled. People's thoughts, feelings, and behavior are all within their control. As Ashleigh Brilliant (1981) said, "We have only two things to worry about, either things will get back to normal, or that they already have."

Studies are needed to understand how laughter works, to determine if it affects the immune system or longevity as suggested, and to measure the significance and efficacy of humor as a therapeutic approach (Roach, 1996). From a scientific perspective, no one has ever explained satisfactorily why humans have the capacity to laugh. Nevertheless, humans do laugh, and laughter appears to have physiological benefits for both nurses and patients.

THE IMPORTANCE OF THE ENVIRONMENT

One way to look at environment (Kayser-Jones, 1989) is to look at the parts that make up the whole of a person's surroundings, such as in a nursing home. The parts include the physical environment, the psychosocial environment, and the organizational environment. One model developed to examine the relationship between the environment and patients with Alzheimer's disease (Hall & Buckwalter, 1987) speculates that as dementia progresses the patient will be more affected by the environment. This idea means that staff personnel and administrators of nursing facilities must look closely at the amount and kind of stimuli and demands that the nursing home environment creates for patients who have Alzheimer's disease.

The physical environment for nursing homes was outlined by the Omnibus Budget Reconciliation Act in 1987. The emphasis was on providing care in a manner and in an environment that would promote the maintenance or enhancement of the quality of life of each resident. The physical environment should support and expand the experience of daily living through contact with food preparation (sounds and smells), a homelike setting for watching television or people, and group settings that encourage socializing (Rader, 1996a).

Nurses should look at the areas in a nursing facility, hospital, or home that make up the physical environment. They should assess the personalization of the immediate patient area, the noise level, the lighting (the average 80-year-old requires three times more light than a 20-year-old does), floor coverings and furniture, safety and security, and activities and stimulation. All these factors play a role in minimizing anxiety related to the physical environment in patients with Alzheimer's disease.

When asked, the elderly say that what makes any environment positive is that they are treated with dignity, respect, and kindness. Therefore, creating a positive psychosocial environment is essential. The psychosocial environment involves staff members' attitudes, communication skills, willingness to nurture healthy interpersonal relationships with demented patients, and behavioral approaches; the structure of activities; an atmosphere of friendliness and caring; family support; and educational services (Rader, 1996a). Staff members' attitudes reflect how they view their jobs and how they value residents and families. How the staff responds to difficult behaviors is the key for demented patients. The staff members at a nursing home should recognize the equality of demented patients and so enable the patients to do as much as possible for themselves.

Adults with dementing illnesses often attempt to avoid situations that make them anxious (Hall & Buckwalter, 1987). Nurses can use a patient's anxiety as a barometer to determine what the patient can handle at any particular time. As anxious behaviors occur, activities can be modified and environmental stimuli simplified until the anxiety disappears.

To provide quality care for demented patients, nurses must be involved in all aspects of the environment—physical, psychosocial, and, most important, organizational. The organizational environment affects the systems that cause residents' behavior. Nursing leaders since Florence Nightingale have emphasized the importance of having the authority to provide good nursing. The organizational environment includes the philosophy of the institution, the policies and procedures, staffing patterns, staff education, and availability of equipment and supplies (Rader, 1996a). A less obvious component of the organizational environment is the structure of the day. Particularly for demented patients, the predictability of the daily schedule makes them feel secure and less fearful.

Nurses have the opportunity to affect the organizational environment for patients with Alzheimer's disease and other dementias. It is critical for nurses to examine each aspect of the environment, physical, psychosocial, and organizational, for clues to patients' unmet needs that may precipitate inappropriate behaviors. Nurses must be involved in all aspects of planning and studying the environment for patients with Alzheimer's disease.

SUMMARY

The focus in caring for patients with Alzheimer's disease and other dementias has often been on the tasks rather than the patients. Several therapeutic approaches can be used to deal with patients' behaviors. These methods try to understand what the behavior means and by doing so how to deal with it. The foundation of what nurses do and how they do it is what they believe, their underlying philosophy. Nurses who think that behavior has meaning will act differently toward patients than will nurses who think things just happen. Therapeutic approaches give nurses a framework for dealing with the erratic behaviors of demented patients.

EXAM QUESTIONS

CHAPTER 3
Questions 21–30

21. Which of the following therapeutic approaches originated because of a need for more interpersonal contact between health care workers and residents in nursing homes?

    A. Reality orientation

    B. Validation therapy

    C. Life review

    D. Individualized care

22. Which of the following is a benefit of reminiscing for demented patients?

    A. It promotes intergenerational understanding.

    B. It does not include discussion of painful memories.

    C. It helps patients keep in touch with their surroundings.

    D. It helps overcome confusion.

23. Which of the following techniques is used in reality orientation for patients who have dementia?

    A. Staff members ignore patients' inappropriate behavior.

    B. Patients are helped to put their lives in a broader perspective.

    C. Use of memory aids such as photographs and calendars is encouraged.

    D. Staff members find familiar coping methods that patients can use again.

24. In which of the following situations would patients with Alzheimer's disease benefit most from reminiscence?

    A. When they understand the guidelines

    B. When they are part of a group

    C. When they have not lost their verbal ability

    D. When they have a good sense of humor

25. Patty Wooten, a critical care nurse, has done research on the use of humor and on:

    A. Caring for patients with Alzheimer's disease

    B. Overcoming burnout in nursing jobs

    C. The relationship between stress and cardiac illnesses

    D. Controlling the values a nurse takes into an ICU

26. Which of the following statements about humor as therapy is correct?

    A. No one can explain why humans laugh.

    B. Most people say more good things than bad things about themselves.

    C. People should not repeat things that poke fun at themselves.

    D. Nurses do not need to worry about the meaning of behaviors.

27. Which of the following is an aspect in a nursing home environment that influences the lives of patients with dementia?

    A. Experience of the staff

    B. Skill of the caregiver

    C. Response of the staff to difficult behaviors

    D. Level of anxiety of the caregivers and of the demented patients

28. Nursing assessment of the psychosocial environment includes evaluation of which of the following?

    A. Staff members' willingness to perform the personal care of demented patients

    B. Staff members' attitudes toward patients with Alzheimer's disease and the patients' families

    C. Staffing patterns

    D. Safety and security

29. What is the most important aspect of the organizational environment of an agency or facility?

    A. Policies and procedures

    B. Activities for patients

    C. Its philosophy

    D. Staff education

30. Which of the following therapeutic approaches would be most helpful during the later stages of Alzheimer's disease?

    A. Validation therapy

    B. Reality orientation

    C. Life review

    D. Humor

CHAPTER 4

NURSING THE WHOLE PERSON

CHAPTER OBJECTIVE

After completing this chapter, the reader will be able to describe the nursing process, including best practice interventions, for multidisciplinary concerns of patients with Alzheimer's disease.

LEARNING OBJECTIVES

1. Define the term best practice intervention.

2. Distinguish interventions to improve communication in patients with Alzheimer's disease.

3. Indicate the prevalence of incontinence in the elderly.

4. Recognize which usually occurs first, bowel or urinary incontinence.

5. Choose examples of functional incontinence.

6. Specify a best practice intervention for preventing increases in incontinence in patients with Alzheimer's disease.

7. Recognize the types of malnutrition in the elderly.

8. Differentiate significant loss of body weight for 1-, 3-, and 6-month periods in the elderly.

9. Indicate the goal of a therapeutic activity program for a patient with dementia.

10. Differentiate religion and spirituality.

INTRODUCTION

What nurses do evolves from the nursing process, the problem-solving process that forms the basis for nurses' actions. Once the problem is clearly delineated, the solutions become evident. The nursing process is holistic and does not represent a simple cause-and-effect relationship. One need or concern affects every other need or problem. The nursing process does not deal simply with the physiological or psychological needs of patients with dementing conditions. Needs are overlapping and involve the whole person.

The term, best practices, is used by surveyors of nursing homes to recognize what works well in a practice setting. Best practices are the interventions or tools suggested and used by practitioners and experts in the care of patients with dementia. This chapter describes the best practice interventions to meet a variety of holistic needs of patients with dementia. The strategies are not all encompassing but are suggestive of what has worked best for others. The chapter discusses what works for communication obstacles; incontinence of bladder and bowel; and nutritional challenges, such as eating and swallowing difficulties, thirst, and weight loss. It also address nurses' role in the use of therapeutic activities and in meeting the spiritual needs of patients with Alzheimer's disease.

COMMUNICATION

Patients with dementia experience life "in the moment," and being in the moment is often the key to communicating with and understanding them. According to the *Male Caregiver's Guidebook,* published by the Alzheimer's Association (1990), communication is the most important quality in enhancing a loving relationship, and lack of communication is most destructive to a loving relationship. These facts are not surprising to family caregivers or nurses. Obstacles to communication when caring for someone with a dementing condition can be difficult, overwhelming, and frustrating.

As Alzheimer's disease progresses, patients become able to speak and understand less and less. Communicating with them poses two problems (Mace & Rabins, 1991). One problem is the difficulty these patients have expressing themselves to others (expressive language); the second is the difficulty they have understanding what others say to them (receptive language).

In the early stages of Alzheimer's disease, the difficulties involve short-term memory loss or simply naming things. Understanding humor, following anything but simple directions, and understanding more complex conversations becomes difficult. Patients may have trouble figuring out what they want to say and take longer to "think" about things. In the middle stages, as the neurological condition progresses, disorientation and confusion increase and increasing difficulty understanding and responding to language can cause withdrawal in social situations. In the latter stages, patients may not speak at all or may use repetitive phrases and are usually extremely disoriented.

Failure to understand what a patient is trying to say or failure to comprehend what is being communicated by the patient can lead to catastrophic reactions (see chapter 5). Some basic principles or strategies can help caregivers communicate.

First, slow down and calm down. A slow, calm approach can defuse a potentially escalating situation. If a patient becomes increasingly restless and agitated while attempting to tell you something, use nonverbal skills to enhance the communication. Look directly at the patient, and maintain good eye contact when speaking. Some patients try to hide their problems with finding the right words by saying, "I don't want to talk about it." Others who have not used curse words in the past may start cursing.

If possible, stay on the same positional level with the patient. If the patient is sitting, you sit; if the patient is standing, you stand. Be certain that your verbal and nonverbal messages match. If a disparity exists, patients with dementia are more likely to respond to the unspoken or nonverbal message. Remain aware of your facial expressions, and be alert to the patient's expressions. Use gestures to help in what you are trying to say. Point at what you are describing in words, or use nonverbal cues such as simulating holding a glass and drinking.

When patients have trouble expressing a wish or explaining what they want, try guessing. This best practice is used creatively and effectively by professional and family caregivers. By slowing down and considering both verbal and nonverbal cues, you may pick up on what the patient is trying to say. Ask if you are guessing correctly. Stay relaxed, and repeat or rephrase what you think is being said. Watch for gestures or signals that you have guessed correctly or incorrectly. Try responding to the underlying meaning of what a confused patient wants rather than to the specific words said (Rader, 1996c). This practice promotes the dignity of the patient and helps isolate and meet unmet needs.

In communicating with a patient with Alzheimer's disease, touch becomes even more meaningful and significant than before (Aspen Reference Group, 1995). As people grow older, they long to be touched by other caring people. When verbal skills are impaired or changed, touch becomes more important. Proper touching includes the following: Before touching a patient, make certain that the patient sees you. Avoid startling with a sudden touch. Touch gradually while looking for a reaction. Notice if the patient pulls away or changes position. This reaction may indicate that the touch is not pleasurable. A light touch is usually considered a stimulant. A firm touch is calming and can be reassuring. Touching is more agreeable on certain areas of the body than on other areas. One area that is easily touched and on which touching is calming is the upper arm between the shoulder and elbow.

Touching patients who have dementia can also produce unexpected reactions. They may become angry or even sexually aroused. This reaction does not mean that you did something wrong. Just distract the patient and remain calm. When the brain is involved, as it is in Alzheimer's disease, misinterpretations occur, so do not avoid touching simply because it might be misunderstood. Touching builds trust and communication and prevents feelings of isolation and loneliness (Gwyther, 1985).

Many nurses and other staff personnel find it distressing when a patient with dementia asks the same question or repeats the same statement over and over again. For example, Mrs. Turner asked repeatedly when her daughter was coming. Staff members would sometimes tell her that her daughter lived out of state and was "just here last month." The question would be repeated in a few minutes. This behavior may be a sign of the fear and insecurity Mrs. Turner is experiencing, or it may simply be an indication that she cannot remember things for even brief periods and does not realize that she received an answer a short time ago (Mace & Rabins, 1991).

For repetitious questioning or statements, several different strategies may work. For some

patients, ignoring the statement or question may work. For others, this strategy makes the situation worse and upsets them. Sometimes distraction helps. Take the patient for a walk or provide a snack or juice. For some patients, rather than answering repeated questions, try reassuring them that everything is fine and that you will take care of things. The meaning behind the repetitive questions or statements may be fear or worry. For example, Mrs. Turner worried that not being in her own home would make her miss her daughter's visit. Remember, though, as with all interventions, what works today, or this morning, may not work the next time; so be flexible.

Being in the moment to communicate with patients with Alzheimer's disease involves the following:

1. Listen to what is said and seek out what is unspoken.

2. Always treat the patient as an adult. Do not talk down.

3. Speak slowly and in a low-pitched voice and identify yourself during each interaction. Do not ask if the patient remembers your name.

4. When you ask a question, wait for an answer. If the patient does not answer, repeat the question. For example, point to the patient's arm and say "Does your arm hurt? Does your arm hurt?"

5. If the patient is stuck for a word, try guessing. Use words, gestures, pictures, pointing, and facial expressions to help.

6. Be consistent, and use simple language. Do not use figures of speech such as "hop into bed" or "let me give you a hand."

When supervising or managing other staff members who communicate with patients with dementia, remind them that verbal and nonverbal strategies can be taught and learned. Some persons seem to have an innate awareness of how to communicate with patients with dementia (Rader, 1996c). Others appear to be incapable of communicating with these patients or unwilling to learn the methods for effective and compassionate communication.

Rader speculates that some staff members may lack insight into how their behaviors affect others. These staff members refuse to alter their style to accommodate others and continue to talk loudly and hurry through tasks in an abrupt and controlling manner. Any staff member who continues to behave in this manner after documented evaluations and ongoing inservice training should be informed that he or she is unsuited for working with patients with dementia and should be dismissed from the staff. As Rader (1996c) states, "To continue to employ staff members who have consistently poor psychosocial skills…creates more work for others and severely limits quality of life" (p. 195). Nurses who supervise and manage other staff members must demonstrate proper communication skills to the staff and then, if necessary, make decisions for the benefit of patients, the persons who live with the signs and symptoms of dementia.

INCONTINENCE

Incontinence occurs in 15–30% of the elderly in the community and in up to 50% of the elderly who are institutionalized (Ebersole & Hess, 1994). These percentages are much higher for patients with dementia and are a significant factor in institutionalizing patients with Alzheimer's disease. Family and professional caregivers react strongly to toileting problems as incontinence develops (Hutchinson, Leger-Krall & Skodol Wilson, 1996).

When incontinence develops in patients with Alzheimer's disease, urinary problems usually occur before bowel problems. Functional incontinence is the term used to describe the incontinence that most often occurs during the course of Alzheimer's disease. This type of incontinence is related to pathophysiological changes that affect emptying the bladder. Urine is lost because the patient is unaware of the need to urinate or cannot reach a toilet because of immobility. Medications and the environment can also cause functional incontinence. Everyone urinates more often as he or she becomes older, but incontinence should be managed (Gwyther, 1985). Managing incontinence involves looking for the underlying causes and attempting corrective action.

The 1991 update of the Omnibus Budget Reconciliation Act mandated that residents in nursing homes must be assessed, and a plan of care developed. Urinary incontinence was one of the major issues focused on as clinical practice guidelines evolved. In patients with functional incontinence such as occurs in Alzheimer's disease, efforts must be made to implement a toileting program (U.S. Department of Health and Human Services, 1992).

In the early stages of Alzheimer's disease, incontinence is not a normal part of the disease. It may be due to other problems that should be detected and treated. Possible problems include the following:

- Urinary tract infections.

- Other acute illnesses.

- Fluids such as coffee, tea, or colas that act as diuretics

- Fecal impaction: As the urethra is pinched off by the stool, bladder control is lost, and urine is released in spurts and trickles to prevent rupture.

- Dehydration: Not enough fluids can lead to overconcentrated urine that irritates the bladder and causes difficulties in bladder control.

- Out-of-control chronic illness such as diabetes or congestive heart failure.

- Enlarged prostate.

- Inability to reach the toilet independently.

- Drugs: Use of sedatives, hypnotics, antidepressants, anticholinergics, diuretics, and antianxiety agents should be evaluated. Drugs that diminish a person's ability to feel body sensations, such as the urge to urinate, are often drugs that calm or sedate.

Excellent urinary and bowel incontinence assessment forms are available and can easily be ordered and adopted. However, each nurse should seek out and implement the assessment format that works best for him or her, within the limits of the employing agency or facility. Interestingly, in practice, bowel incontinence is not considered as much of a problem as urinary incontinence is, because bowel elimination only occurs every 1–2 days (Hutchinson et al, 1996). The best way to treat urinary incontinence is to detect the underlying cause, and then, if possible, treat the cause. A urinary tract infection or pneumonia can occur concurrently with urinary incontinence.

As problems occur with incontinence, families and residential caregivers begin to look for cues from the patient so that they will recognize when toileting is needed. Cues may be verbal or nonverbal, and their presence should be part of the assessment for incontinence. Talk to the family, if the patient is at home, or to the hands-on caregiver to find out how the patient signals the need to go to the bathroom. Cues may be behavioral, such as becoming restless or fidgety; trying to get up or, at night, trying to get up without help; or wandering at night. Experienced staff and caregivers can tell when toileting is needed by "reading" the eyes or facial expressions of patients.

Assessment of each patient's pattern of urinary incontinence is critical. The pattern can be assessed during a 3- to 4-day period. The patient is monitored every 1–2 hr for incidents of incontinence or voiding, and the findings are recorded. The record,

at the end of the assessment period, shows when the patient should be toileted on the basis of the patient's individual schedule, not some preestablished idea of toileting every 2 hr. For example, Mr. Jackson needs to urinate several times in the morning and then only once in the afternoon and once after the evening meal. He does not like to get out of bed at night, so he will need to have a urinal placed by his bed at night where he can see it. Perhaps, Mr. Jackson will need to be reminded occasionally what the urinal is for. The key to a toileting program is to individualize it to the patient's schedule for urinating.

Maintaining dignity and privacy are two of the major issues related to incontinence. Best practices include being discreet when talking to a patient about toileting. Whispering when discussing toileting needs, although acting natural, and avoiding embarrassment are keys. Another best practice involves not using pads for incontinence when the person is only intermittently incontinent. Apparently, simply applying the brief or pad encourages the patient to rely on the pad and lose toileting abilities and is also humiliating and degrading. In addition, staff members seem to attend first to patients who do not wear pads or briefs for incontinence.

Patients with dementia require both physical and cognitive assistance to meet their toileting needs. Factors that affect toileting programs in a facility are the size and weight of the patient and his or her need for assistive devices (Hutchinson et al, 1996). Toileting becomes more time-consuming and potentially dangerous with larger or heavier patients. Practices for toileting that include recognition of physical and cognitive needs include the following (Hutchinson et al, 1996):

- Follow routines that fit the patient's schedule.

- Have the patient drink six to eight glasses of fluids each day.

- Be observant and read verbal and behavioral cues.

- Respond to the cues.

- Communicate regularly with the patient's family members or other caregivers as conditions change.

- Be consistent and make toileting each patient a priority. When professional or family caregivers get busy, the first routine to suffer is toileting.

The goal of any program for patients with Alzheimer's disease or other dementia is to encourage the patients' functional abilities as long as possible and to enhance the quality of their life. Consider the following example: Recently, in a nursing facility, an elderly man with dementia, Mr. Sloan, was observed in the afternoon trying to crawl over his bed rails. His sheets were wet from top to bottom. When a nurse approached, Mr. Sloan explained, although confused, that he had finished his nap and wanted to get up now. He also pointed to his wet sheets and said, "I sweat a lot when I sleep." Although this gentleman could not make many of his needs known verbally at this point, he wanted to retain his sense of personal dignity by explaining the wet bed as he wished the nurse to see it. This knowledge underscores the care and services that nurses provide to manage the needs of patients with dementia who are incontinent.

NUTRITION

Food is more than just something to eat. Food turns a meal into a sensory and social transaction that brings quality to the life of any person and especially one with dementia. According to estimates, 85% of elderly patients in either nursing homes or hospitals are malnourished. No one is deliberately starving the frail elderly, but they may forget to eat or be too tired to eat without some kind of intervention. Common problems of the elderly can be due to not eating or to malnourishment. These include fatigue; increasing confusion; greater risk of infections; skin breakdown due to thinning, shearing, or tearing; and poor wound healing.

Protein-calorie malnutrition, caused by famine in developing countries, can occur in institutionalized elderly people who take in too little protein or too few calories or both for too long (Yen, 1989). All nutritional deficiencies are less easily detected in the elderly than in younger persons. Diseases and the medications used to treat them, plus the process of aging itself, can modify biochemical standards used to assess nutritional status. For instance, kidney or liver damage can potentially affect albumin levels and diminish the value of albumin assays as a tool.

Change in body weight, loss or gain, is the most significant indicator of nutritional status in the elderly, particularly in patients with dementia who wander. In one study (Thomas, 1995), loss of weight was judged to be a substantial concern for patients with Alzheimer's disease, who lost 21% more weight than nondemented patients. Calorie depletion is high during wandering, and patients who wander are less able than other patients to sit still long enough to eat a meal. Thus, weight loss is critical (Singh, Mulley, & Losowsky, 1988).

According to the HCFA, weight loss in nursing home residents is significant when it reaches the following levels of loss: 5.0% of body weight in 1 month, 7.5% in 3 months, and 10.0% in 6 months. These losses may indicate changes in diet, activity, metabolism, or ability to eat or swallow the food being served. Obesity can also be a sign of malnutrition. Weight that is 20% above or 10% percent below desirable values (for height) may be a sign of poor nutritional outcomes.

As Alzheimer's disease progresses, the need for assessment of nutritional status and for assistance with eating increases. Nutritional assessment includes keeping a diary of actual food intake, a weight history (including the patient's previous usual body weight, not just weight related to height), and monitoring weight and height during a specified interval. For example, Mr. Wheeler was 6 ft (1.8 m) tall and weighed 155 lb (70 kg) at the time of his assessment. Conversations with his wife revealed that although this weight was below the norm for his height, he had weighed between 155 and 165 lb (70–75 kg) for the previous 15 years, making this weight his usual body weight.

In clinical settings, the serum level of albumin is a useful indicator of a patient's protein status; less than 2.8 g/100 ml is considered severe protein depletion (Ross Laboratories, 1988). Although hemoglobin and hematocrit levels are used to measure iron status, they are also useful indicators of anemia caused by folate or protein deficiency. Hemoglobin levels less than 12 g/dl and hematocrit values less than 0.35 indicate severe anemia, which is more common in women than in men among the elderly. These measures do not present a complete nutritional picture, but they are easy to evaluate, and if a specific nutrient deficiency is suspected, further studies can be done. Because patients with Alzheimer's disease are at high risk for nutritional deficiencies, additional evaluation by a registered dietitian may be indicated.

Adequate intake of fluid is also important in patients with dementia. Fluids should be offered often during the day, because active patients with dementia may forget to drink. Hyperorality is common in Alzheimer's disease. Patients with this condition place objects of all kinds in their mouth, such as beads, flowers, and even hearing aides, and may swallow the objects. These patients should be checked often for foreign objects in the mouth or throat.

The methods use to administer fluids to patients in a hospital or nursing home can be a problem. Pitchers or jugs at the bedside are inconvenient and are often too heavy or bulky for a frail elderly person to handle. This method of providing fluids is also not the one most people use. Some nursing facilities are now setting up systems of best practice to offer and give fluids in ways that more closely resemble how most people get fluids at home and at work.

As patients' ability to perform the activities involved in eating declines, supervision of eating and reassessment are necessary. Patients in the advanced stages of Alzheimer's disease have difficulty remembering the steps needed to bring food to the mouth, chew it, and swallow (Wykle & Morris, 1994). Attention to food preferences is critical in revitalizing the appetite and eating skills. Overeating, not eating at all, or taking food from others is not uncommon. Patients with dementia may have delusions about food and eating, including fears related to shapes and consistencies, and nurses must be aware and tolerant. Caregivers should watch for signs of depression in patients with dementia, because depression can affect appetite. Loss of appetite can be due to medical causes of anorexia, such as dental problems and nausea (Stewart, 1996).

Self-care in nutrition is the goal for as long as possible. Self-feeding can be encouraged by honoring food preferences and by providing finger foods that are truly finger foods, not mashed potatoes eaten with the hands. Avoid restrictive diets. Do not expect "proper" eating. If a patient who wants to eat dessert first, allow the patient to do so. Emphasize high-calorie foods that are nutrient dense (more nutrients in a smaller amount of food, such as a "super cereal"). Encourage patients to eat at their own pace, and provide one-on-one supervision if necessary. Try small feedings.

Because patients with Alzheimer's cannot realistically perceive the environment, some modifications must be made. To prevent burning, be sure food is not too hot to put in the mouth. Food that is too hot is a more common problem in the home. Provide a quiet, well-lighted setting for meals. Fewer distractions mean more food may be consumed. Because darker colors are often perceived as a "stop" signal, use white or light-colored plates and bowls with little or no pattern. Other suggestions for meal preparation and serving include the following:

- Debone meats.

- Do not use individual packets for condiments or small containers of cream or butter.

- Pour milk into a glass rather than leaving it in the carton, and do not provide straws unless specifically indicated.

- Serve rolls rather than slices of bread.

- Serve soup in cups rather than in bowls.

- Unwrap napkins if they are wrapped in plastic.

In later stages of the disease, the following practices are recommended:

- Serve decaffeinated coffee unless the patient specifically requests regular coffee.

- Use forks and spoons only. For patients in later stages, use spoons only and cut all food before presenting it to the patient.

An early sign of being unable to chew or swallow is the holding of food in the mouth. Pureed or chopped food may help, but in the advanced stages of Alzheimer's disease, patients may lose the ability to chew or swallow completely. At this time, critical decisions must be made about providing nourishment through feeding tubes. Patience, skill, consistency, and knowing the patient's needs can have a significant impact on how soon, or if, these decisions must be made.

THERAPEUTIC ACTIVITY

Therapeutic activities are used to prevent behavioral problems in patients with Alzheimer's disease while enabling the patients to feel useful rather than helpless (Mace, 1984). Therapeutic activities are what people do to search for meaning and purpose in life. In fact, humans and animals will create activity when none exists. One goal of the Omnibus Budget Reconciliation Act was to maintain quality of life and pleasurable activity for patients with dementia. The goal of an activity program for such patients is to reduce feelings of failure and provide a feeling of belonging while enhancing self-esteem (Weaver, 1996). This goal is reached by having insight into the special emotional needs of each patient with Alzheimer's disease, by exploring the patient's strengths, and by attempting to understand what activities can provide satisfaction and meaning to that patient. A distinction should be made between "events" that occur, for instance in a nursing facility, and therapeutic activities. Bringing in a barbershop quartet or someone to sing Christmas carols or hymns or play the accordion is not a therapeutic activity unless the event has meaning for the patients present. Nurses must have an awareness of each patient and his or her unique needs.

Persons with dementia need a balance between rest and activity (Hall & Buckwalter, 1987), and nurses have always played a major role in determining the ratio of activity to rest. By recognizing the therapeutic value of patients' self-care, nurses participate in exercise and activity programs in patients' homes and in other practice settings.

To meet the needs of individual patients, therapeutic activity programs include the following types of activities (Helm & Wekstein, 1991):

- **Mental stimulation:** Reading, talking, reminiscing.

- **Socialization:** Discussions, mealtime, any group or gathering.

- **Creative activity:** Crafts, needlework, story-telling.

- **Productive activity:** Building something, providing a service to another.

- **Emotionally supportive activity:** Support group, one-to-one attention.

- **Physical activity:** Walking, exercise, movement to music.

- **Personal care:** Bathing, dressing, eating.

Observant nurses can notice when a patient is becoming anxious and can respond with an appropriate therapeutic activity. Many traditional nursing interventions encompass the benefits and characteristics of therapeutic activity.

Any of these activities can be provided by nurses or can be taught to other staff members or caregivers in settings that do not have specific people to handle therapeutic activities. The environment for therapeutic activity for patients with Alzheimer's disease should be failure-free, have limited goals, and provide structure. The key is that the activity has meaning for the individual patient and provides feelings of increased success and self-esteem.

SPIRITUAL NEEDS

Albert Einstein viewed religion and spirituality as follows: "My religion consists of a humble admiration of the illimitable superior spirit who reveals himself in the slight details we are able to perceive with our frail and feeble mind." Nurses have often assumed that a person's spiritual needs are the same as religious preferences, affiliations, rites, or rituals. Religion can be defined as a system of beliefs and formal practices that are practiced individually or in a community group to provide focus and meaning to life, understand death, and maintain hope for the future (Sullivan, Smidt-Jernstrom, & Rader, 1996). Religion is only one aspect of spirituality.

Spirituality is a much broader term and reflects the individuality of each person's beliefs about relationships, love and intimacy, forgiveness, hopes for the future, and methods of making peace with the past.

Nurses may try to avoid dealing with the spiritual needs of a patient with Alzheimer's disease because they think the needs are too personal or fear they could not recognize spiritual needs and communicate with patients with dementia. The following may be indicators of unmet spiritual needs in an elderly person (Sullivan et al, 1996):

- Fear or anxiety

- Anger or depression

- Guilt

- Grief

- Regret

- Loneliness

- Separation or isolation

- Lack of positive self-image

- Need for reconciliation

- Lack of self-identity

- Alienation

- Questions about the meaning of life

- A sense of unfinished business

Living with Alzheimer's disease means living in a world of fragments. Things do not seem connected. Patients may ask, What am I doing here? What am I going to do next? They may search for wholeness, old identity, long-dead family members, control of familiar ground, or some kind of foundation to make sense of what is happening (Gwyther, 1995). Moving into a nursing home can intensify feelings of isolation and loss of identity and induce feelings about the lack of privacy in a group setting.

Patients spiritual status for unmet needs are assessed through informal, unstructured interviews (see chapter 1 for techniques for interviewing patients with dementia). The nonverbal behavior of the interviewer helps to set up an open, friendly atmosphere in which assessments can be conducted. The interview should determine what the patient's religious background is, what needs are met through the patient's spirituality, and how the spirituality is expressed—through community worship, music, nature, other people such as family, or private prayer. It may be useful to guess at the need that lies behind unknown behaviors after exploring spiritual or religious background with the patient and his or her family.

When a need has been recognized, several actions can be attempted to help patients with Alzheimer's disease meet spiritual needs:

- Offer a supportive presence. Focus on one-to-one visits, involve clergy if possible. Help clergy or church visitors understand that being in the moment with a patient with dementia is more important than a religious discussion. Shared activities can be substituted for limited conversation.

- Share in prayers, scripture readings, or other inspirational readings such as Guideposts. Many patients can read words long after the meaning of the words is lost. Reading is an adult, dignified activity that can be shared and pleasurable. Prayer can work for people because it is thought that God listens and does not give advice. Patients with Alzheimer's disease may gain sense of peace from daily devotions, as may family caregivers.

- Suggest attendance at religious services or worship. Give patients with Alzheimer's disease an opportunity to not fail in giving as well as in receiving. Ask how situations were handled in the past in their community church. Encourage clergy to include sacramental rites such as anointing or healing, if appropriate.

Interventions to meet spiritual needs should be comforting and reassuring to patients and uphold their belief systems. Although many patients with dementia cannot express appreciation or even recognize what their spirituality meant to them in the past, they may be helped by the regular, calm presence of someone who cares about them.

EXAM QUESTIONS

CHAPTER 4
Questions 31–40

31. When a nurse uses a best practice intervention, he or she is doing which of the following?

    A. Interpreting what the patient's problem is

    B. Trying different approaches until one works best

    C. Using the strategies that experts and practitioners have suggested

    D. Scanning all possible interventions for the best one

32. Which of the following is a best practice intervention to aid communication?

    A. Guessing what is being expressed

    B. Speaking more quickly to avoid distractions

    C. Not touching patients with Alzheimer's disease to avoid startling them

    D. Ignoring repeated questions

33. What percent of the elderly in the community experience incontinence?

    A. 60–75

    B. 35–50

    C. 15–30

    D. 5–10

34. Which of the following statements most accurately reflects the relationship between incontinence, Alzheimer's disease, and aging?

    A. Frequency of urination decreases as a person ages.

    B. In the early stages of Alzheimer's disease, incontinence is a normal part of the disease.

    C. Medications are rarely the cause of incontinence.

    D. If incontinence develops, urinary problems usually happen before bowel problems do.

35. Functional incontinence in patients with Alzheimer's disease is related to which of the following?

    A. Loss of bladder function

    B. Pathophysiological changes that make the patient unaware of the need to urinate or unable to reach the toilet

    C. Changes in the ability to ask for help

    D. Apathy of staff members or caregivers

36. Which of the following is a best practice intervention for preventing of increased incontinence?

    A. Place all patients on a 2-hr toileting schedule.

    B. Do not use pads for incontinence if the patient is only intermittently incontinent.

    C. When caregivers are busy, use incontinent briefs to prevent accidents.

    D. Try not to read too much into nonverbal language about toileting.

37. What is the most common type of malnutrition in the institutionalized elderly?

    A. Protein-calorie

    B. Non–nutrient-dense

    C. Carbohydrate

    D. Muscle-sparing

38. According to the standards of the Health Care Financing Administration, what is a significant weight loss for an elderly person in 6 months?

    A. 5 lb (2.3 kg)

    B. 10 lb (4.5 kg)

    C. 5% of body weight

    D. 10% of body weight

39. What is the goal of a therapeutic activity program for a patient with dementia?

    A. To decrease feelings of failure and provide feelings of belonging while enhancing self-esteem of the person

    B. To provide celebrations as holidays occur

    C. To involve the community in providing entertainment for patients with dementia

    D. To encourage increases in eye-hand coordination by use of arts and crafts

40. Which of the following statements best reflects the difference between religion and spirituality?

    A. Spiritual needs are easier to recognize in a person with Alzheimer's disease than religious needs.

    B. Religion is the system of beliefs and practices that give meaning to life while spirituality is more comprehensive.

    C. Spiritual needs can be met by caregivers, while religious needs must be met by clergy.

    D. Spirituality is one aspect of religious training.

CHAPTER 5

COMPLEX BEHAVIORS AND THEIR MANAGEMENT

CHAPTER OBJECTIVE

After completing this chapter, the reader will be able to describe the rationale for using alternatives to physical and chemical restraints to manage behaviors and the appropriate nursing management of behaviors that may occur when caring for patients with Alzheimer's disease, including wandering, resisting care, sleeping problems, and catastrophic reactions.

LEARNING OBJECTIVES

1. Recognize the extent of the use of restraints for the hospitalized elderly.

2. Specify the nurse's role in the use of physical restraints.

3. Recognize possible underlying physiological causes of agitation or confusion.

4. Indicate interventions to prevent falls in patients with Alzheimer's disease.

5. Distinguish how the body uses drugs as aging occurs.

6. Recognize side effects of use of psychoactive drugs in the elderly.

7. Recognize four types of wanderers.

8. Indicate appropriate nursing responses for sleep problems in patients with Alzheimer's disease.

9. Indicate appropriate nursing responses for catastrophic reactions in patients with Alzheimer's disease.

INTRODUCTION

Nurses try to manage the symptoms or the signs of Alzheimer's disease that they see. In this situation, managing means to control or direct not only the care required for the manifestations of a condition such as Alzheimer's disease but also how other staff members deal with the signs or symptoms. Managers lead, teach, and show by actions and words how others with less experience or education can manage the signs and symptoms encountered. In an environment in which each person's strengths and uniqueness are supported and needs are met, trust and respect are fostered. This chapter discusses the appropriateness of physical and chemical restraints, which historically were used to manage unwanted or disruptive behaviors. It also suggests interventions for some of the more persistent behaviors, such as wandering, resisting care, sleeping problems, agitation, and catastrophic reactions.

THE USE OF RESTRAINTS

The Omnibus Budget Reconciliation Act of 1987 mandated a drastic reduction in the use of physical and chemical restraints in long-term-care facilities. Use of physical restraints and psychoactive medications can have hazardous and adverse outcomes. Anything that inhibits movement is considered a restraint, including vests, geri-chairs, bars, belts, psychotropic medications, and bed rails that keep a person from getting out of bed *(Table 5-1)*. Loss of autonomy, humiliation, and fear epitomize the experience of being restrained. Other consequences are skin breakdown, incontinence, constipation, fecal impaction, depression, behavioral problems, and decline in function such as decreased mobility. The ultimate consequence is death. When a physically restrained person falls or slips out of a wheelchair, the injuries can be much more serious than a fractured hip.

On any given day, half a million patients are physically restrained in hospitals and nursing homes in the United States, more so than in any other Western country. Most patients who are restrained are older adults (Strumpf, Evans, & Schwartz, 1990). In hospitals, an estimated 13–20% of elderly patients are physically restrained. The rate of use of antipsychotic drugs *(Table 5-2)* in nursing homes has been 20–50%, which reflects the high prevalence of behavioral problems (Ray et al., 1993).

Typically, nurses have initiated the decision to restrain patients. Nurses have considered physical restraints as a protection for patients, and as protection for the nurses from litigation. The risk of falling and the need to protect tubes and intravenous lines are often given as reasons for using physical restraints. Nurses in acute care hospitals have not questioned the use of restraints until recently. One study (Matthiesen, Lamb, McCann, Hollinger-Smith, & Walton, 1996) examined nurses' attitudes to, knowledge of, and practice in the use of physical restraints with older patients in the acute care setting. The findings showed little relationship between a nurses's amount of experience working with elderly persons or education about use of restraints and the inappropriate use of

physical restraints. However, significant differences in practice reflected the standard of care and philosophy of the unit or setting where the nurse was working. This finding points out the importance of role models who can show nurses and other caregivers how to solve problems and examine alternatives to the use of restraints. As role models in hospitals and other clinical settings, nurses will be challenged to provide high-quality, cost-effective care for elderly, particularly demented, patients that emphasizes alternatives to restraints. Doing more with less has become a theme of hospital-based care.

Alternatives to restraints include the following:

- Determine and treat underlying physiological causes of agitation or confusion. A useful mnemonic of possible causes is the **Seven I's** (Stewart, 1995).

  1. *I*atrogenic: Caused by the treatment, for example, an anticholinergic agent or a sedative.

  2. *I*nfection: Most often urinary tract infection or pneumonia.

  3. *I*njury: Such as a fractured hip.

  4. **Exacerbation of a preexisting *I*llness:** Such as diabetes or chronic obstructive pulmonary disease.

  5. **Fecal *I*mpaction.**

  6. *I*nconsistency in the environment: Any major change in routines of mealtimes, bedtimes, and so forth.

  7. *Is the person depressed?*

- Modify the environment to include carpeted floors and lowered beds.

- Use positioning devices such as wedge cushions and other specialty cushions.

- Have a wheelchair or seating assessment done by a physical or an occupational therapist (Jones, 1996). As many as 80% of elderly per-

TABLE 5-1
Restraints: Consumer Information Sheet

WHAT ARE RESTRAINTS?
Physical Restraints: Anything near or on your body which restricts movement or your ability to get to a part of your body. Usually a specialty device is used. Examples include: vest or jacket restraints, waist belts, geri-chairs, hand mitts, lap pillows, etc.
Chemical Restraints: Psychoactive drugs used to treat behavioral symptoms in place of good care.

WHY ARE RESTRAINTS USED?
• Because of the myth that they ensure safety
• As a substitute for adequate numbers or levels of staff
• Facility fear of liability

WHAT ARE THE GOOD OUTCOMES OF RESTRAINT USE?
Physical Restraints: In rare instances a restraint may enable a resident to do more, ex.- a half bed rail may allow a partially paralyzed person to turn over; a seat belt may help double amputees to remember that they cannot walk on missing legs (they may have the feeling that their legs are still there).
Chemical Restraints: A resident's distressing behavioral symptom (ex. depression) might be treated with a psychoactive drug when simple measures, such as increased activities or talking with a social worker, do not work.

WHAT ARE THE *POOR* OUTCOMES OF RESTRAINT USE?
Changes in Body systems include: poor circulation, chronic constipation, incontinence, weak muscles, weakened bone structure, pressure sores, increased agitation, depressed appetite, increased threat of pneumonia, increased urinary infections, death, etc.
Changes in Quality of Life include: reduced social contact, withdrawal from surroundings, loss of autonomy, depression, increased problems with sleep patterns, loss of mobility, etc.

LAWS and REGULATIONS
• The Nursing Home Reform Act of 1987 (NHRA) states the resident has the right to be free from…physical or chemical restraints imposed for purposes of discipline or convenience and not required to treat the resident's medical symptoms.
• The NHRA also includes provisions requiring:
  • quality of care—to prevent poor outcomes of care
  • assessment and care planning—for each individual to attain and maintain her highest level of functioning
  • residents be treated in such a manner and environment to enhance quality of life

UNDERLYING PRINCIPLES FOR REDUCING RESTRAINT USE
Resident Assessment: Assessments gather information about how well residents can take care of themselves and when they need help. They identify strengths and weaknesses, plus lifelong habits, daily routines, etc.
Individualized Care Plan: Based on strengths and weaknesses identified on assessment, a care plan is developed on how staff will meet a resident's individual needs. It should describe what each staff person will do and when it will happen. The care plan is designed at a care-planning conference, attended by staff, residents, and their families. The care plan should change as the resident's needs change.

OPTIONS FOR ACTION TO AVOID RESTRAINT USE
• Training staff to assess and meet an individual resident's needs— hunger, toileting, sleep, thirst, etc.—according to the resident's routine rather than the facility's routine.
• A program of activities enjoyed by the resident, such as exercise, outdoor time, small jobs agreed to and enjoyed by the resident, etc.
• Companionship, including volunteers, family, friends, etc.
• Environmental approaches: such as good lighting; mattress on floor to reduce falls; appropriate, comfortable seating; alarms, etc.

TABLE 5-1
Restraints Consumer Information Sheet *(Continued)*

SPECIFIC PROGRAMS USED FOR REDUCING RESTRAINT USE
- Restorative care including walking, bowel and bladder, independent eating, dressing, bathing programs.
- Wheelchair management program—to assure correct size and optimum condition. Wheelchair is used for mobility, not seating.
- Individualized seating program. Chairs should be tailored, the same as wheelchairs, to individual needs.
- SERVE program (self esteem, relaxation, stretching, range of motion and walking);
- Specialized programs for residents with dementia, designed to increase their quality of life;
- Video visits—videotaped family visits when families live far away;
- Wandering program—to promote safe wandering while preserving the rights of others;
- Preventive program based on knowing the resident—to prevent triggering of aggressive behavioral symptoms and using protective intervention as a last resort.

IMPLEMENTING A PROGRAM FOR DECREASED RESTRAINT USE
- Support and encourage the facility management to care for residents by meeting individualized needs.
- Support and encourage professional caregiving staff to think creatively of new ways to identify and meet residents' needs.
- Education for all staff on each person's role in preventing and decreasing restraint use.
- Allay fears of families who have been taught that residents must be restrained for safety.
- Promote closer involvement of the social worker, activities director, pharmacologist, therapists, volunteers and family.
- Encourage permanent staff assignments and giving staff flexibility to meet residents' individualized needs.

Provided by National Citizens' Coalition for Nursing Home Reform, 1424 16th St., N.W., Ste. 202, Washington, DC 20036; Ph. (202) 332-2275; Fax (202) 332-2949.

---

sons experience problems with their wheelchairs, such as discomfort, restricted mobility, and poor posture (Shaw & Taylor, 1992). The most common observation—and rationale for the eventual use of a restraint—is that the person appears to be "sliding" out of his or her chair. Poorly fitted seating can lead to problems with circulation, gastrointestinal and urinary tract dysfunction, and high blood pressure. Other problems include difficulty with speech, swallowing, chewing, breathing, and productive coughing. Informed nurses can make a preliminary assessment of seating and mobility needs *(Table 5-3)* and share it with a physical or an occupational therapist.

- Use motion-sensors or alerting devices.

- Create a nonslip or nonskid surface to walk on. Often the cheaper products, such as nonslip rug backing, work best. Use a nonslip surface or strips on the floor by the side of the bed to avoid the use of bed rails.

- Increase involvement of the patient in psychosocial structured activities.

- Increase supervision and observation times and make changes in nursing care, such as increases in assistance with toileting and ambulation.

- Increase the use of therapeutic touch and active listening by nurses and other caregivers.

It is important to remember that what works today for a patient with Alzheimer's disease or dementia may not work tomorrow. The reality is that continual reassessment is required.

Although great emphasis has been placed on decreasing the use of restraints in health care facilities, one area that has not been addressed is the view of patients' family members. The opinions of patients' family members may be one of the biggest challenges or obstacles to decreasing the use of restraints. Many families believe strongly in the use of restraints to protect their family member from falling or to safeguard the loved one in situa-

TABLE 5-2
Commonly Used Psychoactive Drugs

Antipsychotics (Neuroleptics)

Chlorpromazine (Thorazine)

Fluphenazine (Prolixin)

Haloperidol (Haldol)

Loxapine (Loxitane)

Mesoridazine (Serentil)

Molindone (Moban)

Perphenazine (Trilafon)

Risperidone (Risperdal)

Thioridazine (Mellaril)

Thiothixene (Navane)

Trifluoperazine (Stelazine)

Antidepressants

Amitriptyline (Elavil)

Bupropion (Wellbutrin)

Desipramine (Norpramin)

Doxepin (Sinequan)

Fluoxetine (Prozac)

Imipramine (Tofranil)

Maprotiline (Ludiomil)

Nortriptyline (Pamelor)

Paroxetine (Paxil)

Protriptyline (Vivactil)

Tranylcypromine (Parnate)

Trazodone (Desyrel)

Venlafaxine (Effexor)

Anxiolytics (Antianxiety Agents)

Short-acting Benzodiazapines

Alprazolam (Xanax)

Lorazepam (Ativan)

Oxazepam (Serax)

Long-acting Benzodiazepines

Chlordiazepoxide (Librium)

Clonazepam (Klonopin)

Clorazepate (Tranxene)

Diazepam (Valium)

Halazepam (Paxipam)

Prazepam (Centrax)

Temazepam (Restoril)

tions in which "not enough help" is available. Most family members are not informed that a hospitalized patient is going to be restrained and are not given a specific reason for the restraint or told the potential benefits or risks of using restraints (Kanski et al, 1996). Nurses in each practice setting should determine who is responsible for educating families about the families' legal rights, the benefits and risks of the use of restraints, and the alternatives to restraints.

The best time to discuss the use of restraints is before or at the time of admission. Informal conferences can be held to discuss the relevant issues with other caregivers and patients' families. Nurses should keep communication with patients' families open and should provide family members with information such as reprints of articles with easily understood information on the use of restraints. This information reinforces what nurses are attempting to teach and reassures patients and patients' families that although restraint-free care is not "risk-free," the benefits more often outweigh the physical and emotional problems associated with the use of physical restraints.

Some of the drugs that can be considered chemical or pharmacological restraints are antipsychotics, benzodiazepines, sedatives, hypnotics, and antidepressants (Sloane & Hargett, 1997). Federal regulations for nursing homes define a chemical restraint as a drug that is used for discipline of the patient or for the convenience of staff members and is not required to treat a medical sign or symptom, such as hallucinations or delusions—and then only hallucinations or delusions that have an adverse or frightening effect on the patient. A practical nursing approach to drug therapy, particularly, the use of psychoactive drugs, is the concept of benefit versus risk. This idea helps nurses assess patients' potential drug-related problems and provides a useful framework for discussing drug information with patients' families and others (Todd, 1985).

TABLE 5-3
Assessment for Seating and Mobility

Sitting position: Describe how the person usually sits.
• Slouched?
• Leaning forward?
• Leaning to either side? Which side?
• Head forward?
• Position of legs?
    Legs roll in?
    Legs roll out?
    Legs too high?
    Legs too low?
Walking: Yes or No?
• With assistance?
• How much?
• Uses cane?
    Quad cane?
    Walker?
    Brace?
Wheelchair: Yes or No?
• Transfers self?
• Uses arms?
• Uses legs?
• Electric?

Adapted with permission from Jones, D. (1996). Seating problems in long-term care. In J. Rader & E. Youngquist (Eds.), *Individualized dementia care: Creative, compassionate approaches* (pp. 169–189). New York: Springer.

The usual benefit of using a drug is the drug's therapeutic effect. Defining benefits more broadly can include what the patient or the patient's family sees as the benefit of a particular medication. The discussion of benefits should include a look at all drugs being taken, including over-the-counter or "social" drugs such as alcohol or nicotine. Benefits from the use of psychoactive drugs can include increased appetite, weight gain, decreased agitation, and increased ability to socialize.

All drug therapies have an adverse side. Side effects, toxic effects, idiosyncratic reactions, and allergies are some of the risks to consider. Because the elderly have a higher fat-to-lean ratio, lower concentrations of serum albumin, less total body

water, and slower liver metabolism and renal clearance, they need far lower doses of drugs such as antipsychotics than younger persons do. These drugs are stored in fat, so both therapeutic and side effects last much longer. Another rationale for using smaller doses of an antipsychotic is that the lower concentration of albumin means less drug is protein-bound, so more drug is free to circulate (Strome & Howell, 1991). In the elderly, it is important to "start low and go slow" with doses of antipsychotics. Most elderly patients need only one tenth to one third of the usual adult dose to start.

Adverse side effects of antipsychotic agents include anticholinergic effects such as urinary retention, constipation, blurred vision, dry mouth, and confusion, which is more likely to occur in elderly patients with dementia. Other possible side effects are sedation, orthostatic hypotension, photosensitivity, impaired temperature regulation, and depression. Tardive dyskinesia, a side effect that occurs after long-term use of antipsychotics, is characterized by abnormal, involuntary movements, such as lip smacking and lateral movements of the tongue. Neuroleptic malignant syndrome is a rare, but potentially fatal side effect. This medical emergency is characterized by muscular rigidity, high fever, elevated levels of creatine phosphokinase, unstable blood pressure, and confusion. Management involves treating the signs while stopping the medication. Extrapyramidal side effects of antipsychotics include pseudoparkinsonism and akathisia, in which restless movements can often mimic agitation. The ultimate adverse effects can be falls with fractures, loss of connection with the environment, and eventually a poorer quality of life (Simonson, 1996).

Antipsychotics are not appropriate for the treatment of wandering, restlessness, or dementia. They are useful for the treatment of behaviors that are due to a psychosis-related condition or that become a threat to the patient and a danger to others, including staff members, or interfere with the staff's ability to care for the patient. In these instances, the behaviors must be documented and quantified. The American Society of Consultant Pharmacists (cited in Wachter, 1996) has made recommendations for the appropriate use of antipsychotics in long-term-care settings.

1. Use one-time-only dosing of antipsychotics for acute situations and avoid as-needed orders.

2. Set specific criteria for periodic reevaluations of the need for the antipsychotic, and titrate the dose down to the minimum dose for the shortest time span.

3. Encourage the patient's family and others affected by the patient's behavior to become more informed, and improve communication and educational opportunities.

By education and clinical practice, nurses are equipped to detect and assess changes in physical and mental functioning. Knowledge of the risks versus the benefits of psychoactive drugs and changes in the pharmacokinetics of the elderly can enable nurses to recognize actual and potential problems and intervene quickly and effectively. The reality is that other forms of management for behavioral problems should be tried before any physical or chemical restraints are considered.

WANDERING

Wandering occurs in as many as two thirds of patients with dementia (Stewart, 1995). Patients with Alzheimer's disease or dementia who wander away from home cause tremendous stress to their families. The wandering can result in serious injury to the patient and lead to placement in a nursing home. Thomas (1995) defined wandering as "a purposeful behavior that attempts to fulfill a particular need (from the context of the wanderer), is initiated by a cognitively impaired and disoriented individual and is characterized by excessive ambu-

lation that often leads to safety and/or nuisance related problems."

Although nurses may want to discourage wandering because of concerns about fatigue, physical pain, or extreme use of caloric intake, wandering has some apparent benefits (Heim, 1986). These include stimulation of circulation and oxygenation, promotion of exercise, and decreases in contractures. The goal of nursing management then is to maintain a safe level of wandering without putting patients with dementia at great risk.

There seem to be four types of wanderers (Hussain, 1985):

1. **Exit seekers:** Whether looking for someone or something, the person wants to leave the building.

2. **Akathesiacs:** The person is restless, pacing, and agitated. The wandering may be due to prolonged use of psychotropic drugs.

3. **Self-stimulators:** The person wants to stimulate himself or herself by touching walls or doors or turning door knobs.

4. **Modelers:** The person follows others around and copies what they do by going where they go.

Wandering may be related to stress, boredom, feeling lost, acting out past work roles, being in pain, or needing to urinate.

The primary step in managing wandering is to determine the underlying cause of the wandering (Coltharp, Richie, & Kaas, 1996). By creating an outline of when (especially time of day) and under what circumstances the wandering occurs, nurses can develop a plan for dealing with the behavior *(Table 5-4)*. Managing the environment is one of the best methods of dealing with wandering. Visual barriers across doorways, on the floor in front of doors, or over doorknobs are effective. Wandering generally does not respond well to drug therapy. Some psychotropic medications make wandering

---

TABLE 5-4
Guidelines for Nursing Management of Wandering

1. Look for the basis of the behavior.

2. Restructure the environment by the use of visual barriers, electronic alerting systems, and visual cuing. Decrease noise and confusion.

3. Encourage interaction with others in areas set aside for socialization.

4. Use activities that promote self-esteem, such as a collage of pictures supplied by the patient's family or an audiotape or videotape.

5. Go out with the patient—through one door and back in another—or take him or her for a walk.

6. Provide regular exercise and diversion.

7. Use simple language and simple signs to provide cues.

8. Monitor often for physiological needs and meet the patient's need to feel secure and safe.

9. Have patients with dementia wear some type of identification, and alert all staff (or neighbors if at home) to patients who wander.

Adapted with permission from Coltharp, W., Richie, M., & Kaas, M. (1996). Wandering. *Journal of Gerontological Nursing, 22*(11), 5–10.

---

worse by stimulating akathisia.

RESISTING CARE

Caregivers, whether professional or family, often must help patients with dementia eat, bathe, use the toilet, dress, and take medication. Providing this assistance can be a source of stress for the caregiver. Coltharp et al. (1996) formulated a definition of resisting care as "any behavior by the individual which prevents or interferes with the nurse (caregiver) performing or assisting with ADLs [activities of daily living], including bathing, eating, toileting, dressing and grooming." Patients with Alzheimer's disease or dementia may angrily object to the assistance, become verbally or physically abusive, hit, slap, bite, scream, run away, argue, or become agitated. As the behavior escalates, mental, emotional, or physical abuse of the patient by the caregiver may occur. If all behavior has meaning, what does this behavior mean?

Consider this example: Mrs. Durning, a 75-year-old woman with dementia, wears glasses and usually wears a favorite yellow sweater with her blouse and slacks. She walks around the nursing unit at Sunnybrook Nursing Home and is often found in the television room on the far side of the residence. She smiles, is friendly, eats well, and enjoys small-group activities. Her caregiver reported that Mrs. Durning appears to get along just fine, until shower time. At this time, she becomes aggressive, loudly objects to being showered, and has hit and slapped some staff members. During the conversation about the shower incidents, the caregiver stated that there was only one nursing assistant that Mrs. Durning liked. This assistant was a woman who worked nights. The assistant never had any trouble with Mrs. Durning. Staff members recognized, with the help of the patient's family, that Mrs. Durning was a morning person and had always been shy, particularly around men. Letting the staff person who had the best relationship with her care for her and honoring her preference for female caregivers were the first steps in managing the behavior.

When a patient refuses to take a bath or a shower, the reason may be that the whole process has become confusing and perplexing. The ability to process incoming stimuli decreases as dementia increases, and the environment outside becomes the only way for the patient to interpret what is happening. The demented patient's perspective might be as follows: A person comes in to see you, removes you from your bed, and takes your clothes off. If you object, you are given a smile and a pat on the arm. Your calls for help are often ignored. Often, in a nursing facility, you are taken down a cold, public hallway, with a thin sheet or blanket covering your most private parts, and taken into a cold, noisy, strange room where all covering is removed.

Many people have never had anyone see them bathe or shower. Bathing and showering are extremely private activities. The bathing process should be individualized to the needs and routines of the patient involved (Rader, 1996a). It is not necessary to bathe every day or to shower or bathe on certain days or at prearranged times. If Mrs. Durning accepted a shower early in the morning from her favorite staff member, she had her shower then. If she refused, staff members altered plans to meet her needs.

The first principle of nursing management of patients who resist help with any activity of daily living is to determine the cause of the problem (assessment). When, where, and how often does the behavior occur? If a physical problem such as pain or constipation is discovered, it should be dealt with first. Nurses should examine their own or staff members' feelings and responses to the situations that occur (Coltharp et al., 1996). The activity that the patient resists should be carried out in a calm, friendly, gentle manner without rush or hurry. For example, the environment for the bath can be altered. Possible changes include covering mirrors; installing grab bars; using a shower or tub seat; avoiding bath oils or bubble bath; and, in general, making the bathroom a gentler, softer, quieter place. In some rare instances, low doses of lorazepam (Ativan) are effective and well tolerated and have minimal side effects when other interventions to decrease resistance have been unsuccessful (Stewart, 1995).

Goals should be realistic. When a patient resists help with dressing, expectations can be modified. Wearing the same clothing 2 days in a row is all right. Removing a patient's soiled clothing from the room at night avoids arguments. If choices are confusing, they should be eliminated. Dressing can be simplified to sturdy, washable clothing with Velcro fastenings.

Resistance to toileting can be met by determining underlying causes such as burning or pain associated with a urinary tract infection. Also, easily pulled on and off pants and slacks can be substituted for ones with complex zippers and buttons. The bathroom and toilet can be marked with signs that cue patients to the use and location of these facilities.

The key to management of resistance to care is to be flexible and imaginative. The trial-and-error method is useful for finding what works. Of course, what works today may not work tomorrow.

As dementing illnesses progress, patients become less able to care for themselves. In the early stages of a dementing condition, patients may be able to cover up for this deficit. However, they still may be unsafe to do manual tasks and need supervision. This situation does not mean that a nurse should do things for patients who are able to dress or bathe themselves. It does mean that nurses should approach the care of patients with dementia in a slow, calm, open manner while taking the time to assess the patients' self-care abilities.

SLEEP DISTURBANCES

Sleep patterns change with aging. Older adults have lighter sleep and awaken more easily because of degenerative changes in the CNS. Nocturia, muscle cramps, and susceptibility to noise interrupt sleep for older persons, who then require more time to return to sleep (Eliopoulis, 1995). Normal sleep is divided into two types: REM and non-REM (Ham & Sloane, 1997). Each night, sleep begins with non-REM sleep, which is followed in about 2 hr by REM sleep that recurs three to four times each night at regular intervals. With age, people have less deep sleep (stage 4 non-REM sleep) and less REM sleep. Patients with Alzheimer's disease have a further reduction in non-REM and REM sleep (Eliopoulis, 1995). Patients with Alzheimer's disease cannot connect the meaning of sleep cues in the environment (e.g., darkness or quiet) to the sleep cycle. Nighttime wandering can be dangerous and puts an added burden on the caregiver, whether at home or in a health care facility.

Sleeplessness is a serious nursing management issue. Attempts to increase a patient's awareness of time, such as reorientation to the time of day with access to daylight, may be helpful. Restricting food or drinks containing caffeine late in the day may also help. A regular exercise and napping schedule during the daytime is beneficial. When putting patients with dementia to bed at night, caregivers should use a night-light and follow an established regular bathroom and bedtime ritual. A commode can be put at the bedside for use during the night. No attempt should be made to keep patients in bed by using bed rails or, at home, placing a chair next to the bed. If the patient awakens because of pain, pain medication can be provided at bedtime.

The most important strategy is to allow patients who wake up to get out of bed if they want to. For example, Mr. Foster went to bed early every evening. He had been a railroad engineer and always had been an early riser. He would wake up at 2 or 2:30 a.m. and want to get up. Staff members would take him to a safe, quiet place near where they worked, give him a snack, and turn on the television or read to him. If necessary, they let him sleep in a recliner chair either in his room or near them. The key is supervision and responding to the individual patient's needs.

When patients with dementia live at home, nurses can help the patients' caregivers make the nights manageable (Adams & Richmond, 1996). The bedtime and bathroom routine, daytime exercise and activities, and elimination of caffeine and alcohol after 5 p.m. are important at home also. In addition, caregivers can help someone with dementia relax by using soft music (of the type the person prefers) and giving the person a massage or back rub at bedtime. Confrontations about bathing and putting on pajamas at bedtime should be avoided.

Caregivers can make the home as safe as possible by lighting the bathroom, keeping the area around the patient's bed cleared, and using nonskid strips by the side of the bed to prevent the patient from falling or slipping when getting up. Caregivers should also block stairs, lock doors and windows, and lock up dangerous items such as knives or scissors. A room monitor may be helpful if the caregiver sleeps in another part of the house. Caregivers at home may need to consider respite or in-home care if sleeping problems persist.

Use of sleeping medications is not particularly effective in patients with dementia. Common side effects of these drugs are unsteady gait, which increases the risk of falling, and incontinence. The antihistamines often present in over-the-counter sleeping medications can cause increases in confusion and anticholinergic effects. The use of sedatives at home may help the caregiver get much needed sleep, but sedatives should be avoided in a health care facility where staff members are available at night to meet the individualized needs of patients' with Alzheimer's disease.

CATASTROPHIC REACTIONS

Becoming overwhelmed and overreacting to a situation leads to what is called a catastrophic reaction. In patients with dementia, catastrophic reactions are characterized by sudden emotional outbursts and feelings of terror related to being overwhelmed, distressed, or confused by situations or by failing (Mace, 1984). During the emotional outburst, the person displays behaviors such as the following:

- Stubbornness
- Being overly critical
- Rapidly changing moods
- Worry and fear
- Anger and suspiciousness
- Excessive crying
- Increasing restlessness, pacing, and wandering
- Striking out (combativeness)

These reactions appear to be set off by inconsequential situations, often related to the inability to do a simple task, such as brushing hair or washing dishes. A sudden increase in catastrophic reactions may be an early indicator of a developing medical problem such as an infection (Rader, 1996a). Catastrophic reactions most often occur in the morning hours in a health care facility, when daily care activities are greatest (Taylor, Ray, & Meador, 1994). At this time, staff members are under pressure to follow a schedule and place more demands on the patients to complete bathing and grooming tasks.

Catastrophic reactions are disturbing and cause stress to caregivers and nursing staff. The best management technique is to try to understand the cause of the behavior and head off the reaction before it occurs. In addition to the communication techniques discussed in chapters 3 and 4, the following strategies may be helpful:

1. Create a no-fail, low-demand environment with a consistent, predictable schedule.

2. Give directions one step at a time, in simple language. Break the tasks down into easy steps and limit choices.

3. Help the patient accept his or her inability to perform a task by staying calm and not becoming irritated or angry at failure to perform a task.

Once the catastrophic reaction is occurring, other strategies may be more helpful:

1. Let the person with the best relationship with the patient respond.

2. Do not ask questions, argue, restrain, or try to reason with an agitated person.

3. Give verbal reassurance that you understand the patient's fear and embarrassment. Use touch if the patient is responsive to it; pat the patient's arm or shoulder and use soothing music.

4. Guide the patient to a quiet place or offer distraction with a conversation or activity.

5. Get other staff members to assist, and, if necessary, get out of range or leave the room. If attempts to divert the reaction are unsuccessful, do not take the outcome personally.

If catastrophic reactions are occurring frequently, caregivers and nurses can keep a log of what happens, when it happens, who was around, and what helps. They can use the data to look for patterns of events or times that may trigger the reaction. After the reaction is over, they should reassure the patient that they recognize that this reaction can be upsetting to the patient as well as to staff members and that they will continue to care for the patient.

SUMMARY

Managing the care for patients with Alzheimer's disease and other dementias is an enormous challenge for health care providers. About 20–80% of all persons who live in nursing homes sometimes behave in ways that cause problems for professional and family caregivers. Effective coping with behavior problems requires that staff members be understanding, flexible, and creative and listen with the "third ear" (Vollen, 1996). Vollen offers a framework, with the mnemonic TIME, for dealing with behaviors by determining these components:

- **Together:** Work together and plan together to get the best results.

- **Investigate:** Explore the causes of the behavior.

- **Measure:** Quantify the occurrences of specific behaviors to picture behavioral patterns.

- **Empathize:** Try to see the behavior from the point of view of the person with dementia.

Behavioral problems encountered with patients with Alzheimer's disease and other dementias include wandering, resisting care, sleep disturbances, and catastrophic reactions. A basic premise for dealing with these problems is that all behavior has meaning. Caregivers and nurses may not understand or recognize the meaning, but it is there. Nurses can encourage behavioral changes by teaching and modeling methods of coping for staff and family caregivers. Continuing to learn and expand the repertoire of management strategies is essential in caring for patients with Alzheimer's disease.

EXAM QUESTIONS

CHAPTER 5
Questions 41–50

41. According to estimates, what percent of hospitalized older adults are physically restrained?

    A. 7–10

    B. 13–20

    C. 25–30

    D. 33–50

42. Which of the following is the most important action for a nurse to take to reduce the use of restraints?

    A. Become a role model.

    B. Advocate to increase staffing.

    C. Encourage using experienced staff members to care for elderly patients.

    D. Assess patients for the underlying cause of disruptive behaviors.

43. Which of the following is a likely physiological cause of agitation or confusion?

    A. Boredom

    B. Sliding out of a wheelchair

    C. Urinary tract infection

    D. Too many activities

44. Which of the following is the best method to keep a patient with Alzheimer's disease from falling when he or she needs to urinate at night?

    A. Use a nonslip surface next to the bed.

    B. Restrict fluid intake after 3:00 p.m.

    C. Provide increasing periods of exercise.

    D. Give the patient a snack when he or she awakes.

45. Which of the following is a change associated with aging that affects how the body uses drugs?

    A. Lower fat-to-lean ratio

    B. More total body water

    C. Faster renal clearance

    D. Lower concentrations of serum albumin

46. In general, the dose of an antipsychotic for an elderly person should be which of the following?

    A. The same as the dose for other adults

    B. More than one half the usual dose

    C. One tenth to one third greater than the usual dose

    D. One tenth to one third of the usual dose for adults

47. What is the first step to take when an elderly patient suddenly becomes overwhelmed and overreacts to a situation?

    A. Put the bed rails up for safety.

    B. Guide the patient to a quiet place or offer distraction.

    C. Determine if the behavior is due to medications the patient is taking.

    D. Give the patient a snack and check his or her blood glucose level.

48. Which of the following side effects is most likely in an 80-year-old patient with dementia who is taking 0.5 mg of haloperidol three times a day?

    A. Lip smacking

    B. High blood pressure

    C. Confusion

    D. Low-grade fever

49. What type of wanderer is a patient who follows staff members around in a nursing home and attempts to go into other patients' rooms when staff go in to provide care?

    A. Exit seeker

    B. Akathesiac

    C. Self-stimulator

    D. Modeler

50. What is the most important nursing intervention in dealing with sleeplessness in patients who have Alzheimer's disease?

    A. Provide a safe environment.

    B. Be flexible about the time of the nightly bedtime.

    C. Restrict daytime napping to the early afternoon hours.

    D. When patients awake during the night, allow them to get up and have a snack and provide them companionship.

BIBLIOGRAPHY

Adams, L., & Richmond, M. (1996). *Tips for caregivers: sleeping through the night* (Rev. ed.). Santa Cruz, CA: Journeyworks Publishing.

Alzheimer's Association. (1990). *Male caregiver's guidebook: Caring for your loved one with Alzheimer's at home*. Des Moines: Author.

American Psychiatric Association. (1994). *Diagnostic and statistical manual of mental disorders* (4th ed.). Washington, DC: Author.

Aspen Reference Group. (1995). *Home care for people with Alzheimer's disease: Communication* [Videotapep]. Rockville MD: Author.

Brackley, M. (1992). A role supplementation group pilot study: A nursing therapy for parental caregivers. *Clinical Nurse Specialist, 6*(1), 14–19.

Brilliant, A. (1981). *I have abandoned my search for truth and am now looking for a good fantasy*. Woodridge Press.

Buckwalter, K. (1993). Segregating the cognitively impaired. In P. Katz, R. Cane, & M. Mezy (Eds.), *Advances in long term care* (pp. 43–60). New York: Springer.

Burns, H., Howard, R., & Pettit, W. (1995). *Alzheimer's disease: A medical companion*. Cambridge, MA: Blackwell Science.

Butler, R. (1963). The life review: An interpretation of reminiscence in the aged. *Psychiatry Journal for the Study of Interpersonal Process, 26*(11), 68–76.

Clinical News. (1996). *American Journal of Nursing, 96*(11), 9.

Coltharp, W., Richie, M., & Kaas, M. (1996). *Wandering. Journal of Gerontological Nursing, 22*(11), 5–10.

Cousins, N. (1989). *Head first: The biology of hope* (pp. 125–153). New York: Dutton.

Deimling, G., & Bass, D. (1986). Symptoms of mental impairment among elderly adults and their effects on family caregivers. *Journal of Gerontology, 41*(6), 778–784.

Dossey, L. (1996). Now you are fit to live: Humor and health. *Alternative Therapies in Health and Medicine, 2*(5), 8–13, 98–100.

Ebersole, P., & Hess, P. (1994). *Toward healthy aging: Human needs and nursing response* (4th ed.). St. Louis: Mosby.

Eliopoulis, C. (1995). *Manual of gerontologic nursing*. St. Louis: Mosby.

Feil, N. (1982). *Validation: The Feil method*. Cleveland: Edward Feil Productions.

Feil, N. (1987). Research support for interventions that restore well-being in late onset demented populations (Abstract). Proceedings of the Third Congress of the International Psychogeriatrics Association, 3:17.

Feil, N. (1994). *The validation breakthrough.* Baltimore: Health Professions Press.

Folstein, M., Folstein, S., & McHugh, P. (1975). Mini-Mental State: A practical method for grading the cognitive state of patients for the clinician. *Journal of Psychiatric Research, 12*(3), 189–198.

Geldmacher, D., & Whitehouse, P. (1996). Evaluation of dementia. *New England Journal of Medicine, 335*(5), 330–335.

Gwyther, L. (1985). *Care of Alzheimer's patients: A manual for nursing home staff.* Durham, NC: American Health Care Association & Alzheimer's Association.

Gwyther, L. (1995). *You are one of us: Successful church/clergy connections to Alzheimer's families.* Durham NC: Duke University Medical Center.

Hall, G., & Buckwalter, K. (1987). Progressively lowered stress threshold: A conceptual model for care of adults with Alzheimer's disease. *Archives of Psychiatric Nursing, 1*(6), 399–407.

Haycox, J. A. (1984). A simple, reliable clinical behavior scale for assessing demented patients. *Journal of Clinical Psychiatry, 45,* 23–24.

Health Care Financing Administration. (1991). *Guide to choosing a nursing home.* Washington, DC: U.S. Government Office Printing.

Health Care Financing Administration. (1995). *Surveyor's guidebook on dementia* (Pub. No. 386-897/33457). Washington, DC: U.S. Government Printing Office.

Heim, K. (1986). Wandering behavior. *Journal of Gerontologic Nursing, 12*(11), 5–7.

Helm, B., & Wekstein, D. (1991). *For those who take care: An Alzheimer's disease training program for nursing assistants.* Lexington KY: University of Kentucky, Alzheimer's Disease Research Center.

Hendric, H. G., Crossett, V. (1990). An overview of depression in the elderly. *Psychiatric Annals, 20,* 64–69.

Heston, L., & White, J. (1991). *The vanishing mind.* New York: W. H. Freeman.

Hussain, R. (1985). Severe behavioral problems. In L. Terri & E. Lewishohon (Eds.), *Geropsychological assessment and treatment* (pp. 121–144). New York: Springer.

Hutchinson, S., Leger-Krall, S., & Skodol Wilson, H. (1996). Toileting: A behavioral challenge in Alzheimer's disease care. *Journal of Gerontological Nursing, 22*(10), 18–27.

Jacob, S. (1991). Support for family caregivers in the community. *Family and Community Health, 14*(1), 16–21.

Jarvik, L. S. (1988). *Parentcare: A commonsense guide for adult children.* New York: Crown.

Jones, D. (1996). Seating problems in long-term care. In J. Rader & E. Youngquist (Eds.), *Individualized dementia care: Creative, compassionate approaches* (pp. 169–189). New York: Springer.

Jones, P., & Martinson, I. (1992). The experience of bereavement in caregivers of family members with Alzheimer's disease. IMAGE: *The Journal of Nursing Scholarship, 24*(3), 172–176.

Kanski, G., Janelli, L., Jones, H., & Kennedy, M. (1996). Family reactions to restraints in an acute care setting. *Journal of Gerontologic Nursing, 22*(6), 17–22.

Kaplan, H., & Sadock, B. (1988). *Synopsis of psychiatry: Behavioral sciences, clinical psychiatry* (6th ed.). Baltimore: Williams & Wilkins.

Kayser-Jones, J. (1989). The environment and quality of care in long-term care institutions. *Nursing and Health Care, 10*(3), 125–130.

Kovach, C., & Henschel, H. (1996). Planning activities for patients with dementia: A descriptive study on a special care unit. *Journal of Gerontological Nursing, 22*(9), 33–38.

Langner, S. (1993). Ways of managing the experience of caregiving to elderly relatives. *Western Journal of Nursing Research, 15*(5), 582–594.

Laurenhue, K. (1996). *Caregiving with humor and creativity.* Seminar presented for the Alzheimer's Association, Fort Myers, FL.

Lindgren, C. (1993). The caregiver career. *IMAGE: The Journal of Nursing Scholarship, 25*(3), 214–219.

Mace, N. (1984). Facets of dementia: Incontinence. *Journal of Gerontologic Nursing, 10,* 32.

Mace, N., & Rabins, P. (1991). *The 36-hour day* (Rev. ed.). Baltimore: Johns Hopkins University Press.

MacKay, S. (1992). Durable power of attorney for health care. *Geriatric Nursing, 34*(1), 99–108.

Matthiesen, V., Lamb, K., McCann, J., Hollinger-Smith, L., & Walton, J. (1996). Hospital nurses views about physical restraints: Use with older patients. *Journal of Gerontologic Nursing, 22*(6), 8–16.

McCullough, P. (1991). Geriatric depression: Atypical presentations, hidden meanings. *Geriatrics, 46*(10), 72–76.

McKenry, L., & Salerna, E. (1989). *Pharmacology in nursing.* St. Louis: Mosby.

McNeil, C. (1995). *Alzheimer's disease: Unraveling the mystery.* Washington, DC: Public Information Office, National Institute of Aging.

Moffat, N. (1994). Strategies of memory therapy. In B. Wilson & N. Moffat (Eds.), *Clinical management of memory problems* (2nd ed.). San Diego: Singular.

Pietrukowicz, M., & Johnson, M. (1991). Using life histories to individualize nursing home staff attitudes towards residents. *The Gerontologist, 31*(1), 102–106.

Pillemer, K., & Suitor, J. J. (1992). Violence and violent feelings: What causes them among family caregivers? *Journal of Gerontology, 47*(4), S165–S172.

Rader, J. (1996a). Assessing the external environment. In J. Rader & E. Youngquist (Eds.), *Individualized dementia care: Creative, compassionate approaches.* New York: Springer.

Rader, J. (1996b). Creating a supportive environment for eliminating restraints. In J. Rader & E. Youngquist (Eds.), *Individualized dementia care: Creative, compassionate approaches.* New York: Springer.

Rader, J. (1996c). Use of skillful, creative psychosocial interventions. In J. Rader & E. Youngquist (Eds.), *Individualized dementia care: Creative, compassionate approaches.* New York: Springer.

Ray, W., Taylor, J., Meador, K., Lichenstein, M., Griffin, M., Fought, R., Adams, M., & Blazer, D. (1993). Reducing antipsychotic drug use in nursing homes: A controlled trial of provider education. *Archives of Internal Medicine, 153,* 713–721.

Reisberg, B., Ferris, S. H., Leon, M. J., & Crook, T. (1982). The Global Deterioration Scale for assessment of primary degenerative dementia. *American Journal of Psychiatry, 139,* 1136–1139.

Rice, D., Fox, P., & Max, W. (1993). The economic burden of Alzheimer's disease care. *Health Affairs, 12*(2), 164–176.

Roach, M. (1996, September). The laughing clubs of India. *Health,* pp. 93–97.

Ross Laboratories. (1988). *Nutritional assessment: What is it? How is it used?* Columbus, OH: Author.

Sayles-Cross, S. (1993). Perceptions of familial caregivers of adults. *IMAGE: The Journal of Nursing Scholarship, 25*(2), 88–92.

Shaw, C., & Taylor, S. (1992). A survey of wheelchair seating problems of the institutionalized elderly. *Assistive Technology, 3*(1), 5–10.

Simonson, W. (1996). Using psychoactive medications. In J. Rader & E. Youngquist (Eds.), *Individualized dementia care: Creative, compassionate approaches.* New York: Springer.

Singh, S., Mulley, G., & Losowsky, M. (1988). Why are Alzheimer's patients thin? *Age and Ageing, 17,* 21–28.

Sloane, P., & Hargett, F. (1997). Institutionalized care. In R. Ham & P. Sloane (Eds.), *Primary care geriatrics: A case-based approach.* St. Louis: Mosby.

Staab, A. S., & Lyles, M. F. (1990). *Manual of geriatric nursing.* Glenview, IL: Scott, Foresman/Little, Brown Higher Education.

Stewart, J. (1995). Management of problems in the demented patient. *American Academy of Family Physicians, 52*(8), 2311–2318.

Stewart, J. (1996, August). *Psychiatric and behavioral problems in dementia.* Paper presented at the meeting of the Florida Health Care Association, Orlando, FL.

Strome, T., & Howell, T. (1991). How antipsychotics affect the elderly. *American Journal of Nursing, 91*(5), 46–49.

Strumpf, N., Evans, L., & Schwartz, D. (1990). Physical restraint of the elderly. In C. Chenitz, S. Stone, & S. Salesky (Eds), *The clinical practice of gerontological nursing.* Philadelphia: Saunders.

Sullivan, M., Smidt-Jernstrom, K., & Rader, J. (1996). In J. Rader & E. Youngquist (Eds.), *Individualized dementia care: Creative, compassionate approaches.* New York: Springer.

Taylor, J., Ray, W., & Meador, K. (1994). *Managing behavior symptoms in nursing home residents: A manual for nursing staff.* Vanderbilt, TN: Vanderbilt University School of Medicine, Department of Preventive Medicine.

Thomas, D. (1995). Wandering: A proposed definition. *Journal of Gerontological Nursing, 21*(9), 35–44.

Todd, B. (1986). Drugs and the elderly: When the benefits outweigh the risks. *Geriatric Nursing, 7,* 212, 222.

U.S. Department of Health and Human Services. (1992). *Urinary incontinence in adults: Clinical practice guidelines* (AHCPR Pub. No. 92-0038). Rockville, MD: Author.

Vollen, K. (1996). Coping with difficult behaviors takes TIME. *Journal of Gerontological Nursing, 22*(8), 22–26.

Wachter, A. (1996, November). Rethinking psychotropics. *Contemporary Long Term Care,* p. 70H.

Weaver, D. (1996). Activity interventions. In J. Rader & E. Youngquist (Eds.), *Individualized dementia care: Creative, compassionate approaches.* New York: Springer.

Wilson, B., & Moffat, N. (1994). The development of group memory therapy. In B. Wilson & N. Moffat (Eds.), *Clinical management of memory problems* (2nd ed.). San Diego: Singular.

Wooten, P. (1996). Humor: An antidote for stress. *Holistic Nursing Practice, 10*(2), 49–56.

Wykle, M., & Morris, D. (1994). Nursing care in Alzheimer's disease. *Clinics in Geriatric Medicine, 10*(2), 351–360.

Yen, P. K. (1989). Nutrition: The picture of malnutrition. *Geriatric Nursing, 10*(3), 159.

INDEX

PRETEST KEY

1. C   Chapter 1
2. D   Chapter 1
3. C   Chapter 2
4. A   Chapter 2
5. B   Chapter 3
6. D   Chapter 3
7. B   Chapter 4
8. C   Chapter 4
9. D   Chapter 5
10. B   Chapter 5